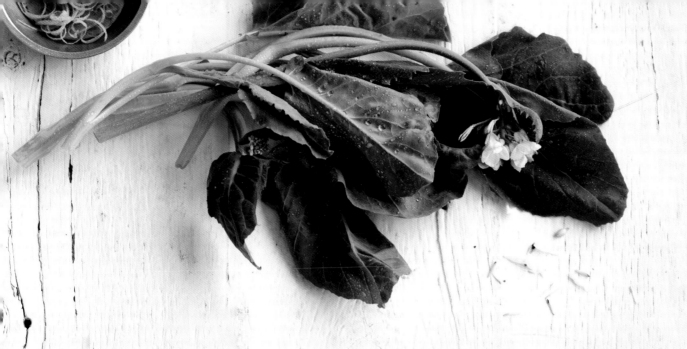

EATING WELL
with diabetes

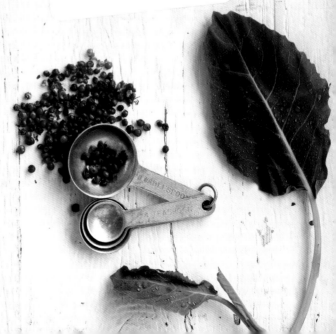

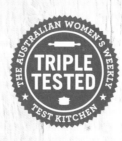

THE AUSTRALIAN WOMEN'S WEEKLY
TRIPLE TESTED
TEST KITCHEN

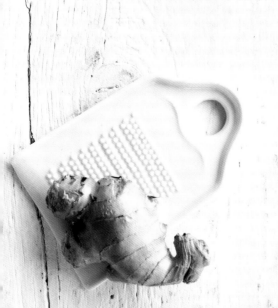

PUBLISHED IN 2015 BY BOUNTY BOOKS BASED ON MATERIALS LICENSED TO IT BY
BAUER MEDIA BOOKS, AUSTRALIA

Bauer Media Books are published by
Bauer Media Pty Limited, 54 Park St, Sydney;
GPO Box 4088, Sydney, NSW 2001, Australia.
phone +61 2 9282 8618; fax +61 2 9126 3702
www.awwcookbooks.com.au

BAUER MEDIA BOOKS
Publisher Jo Runciman
Editorial & food director Pamela Clark
Director of sales, marketing & rights Brian Cearnes
Art director Hannah Blackmore
Designer Jeannel Cunanan
Senoir editor Wendy Bryant
Food editor Emma Braz
Operations manager David Scotto

Printed in China with 1010 Printing Asia Limited

Published and distributed in the United Kingdom by
Bounty Books, a division of
Octopus Publishing Group Ltd

Carmelite House
50 Victoria Embankment
London, EC4Y 0DZ
United Kingdom
info@octopus-publishing.co.uk;
www.octopusbooks.co.uk

International foreign language rights,
Brian Cearnes, Bauer Media Books
bcearnes@bauer-media.com.au

**A catalogue record for this book is available from
the British Library.**
ISBN: 978-0-7537-2994-6
© Bauer Media Pty Limited 2015
ABN 18 053 273 546

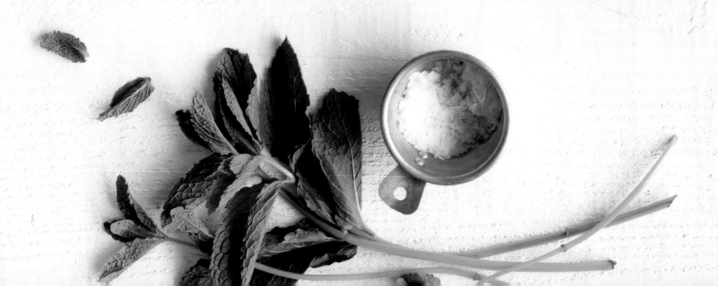

THE AUSTRALIAN
Women's Weekly

EATING WELL
with diabetes

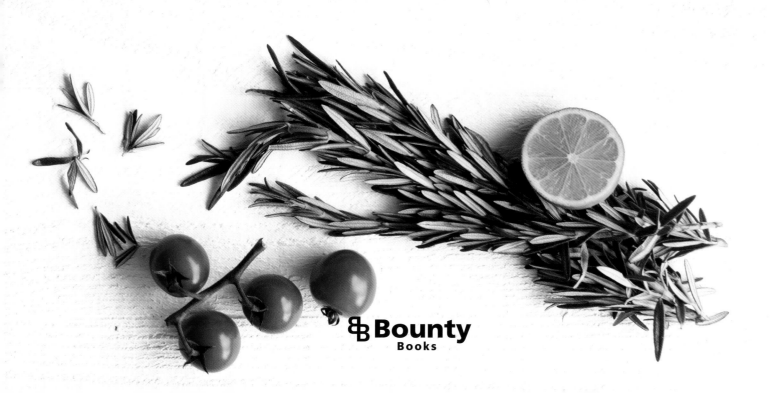

Bounty
Books

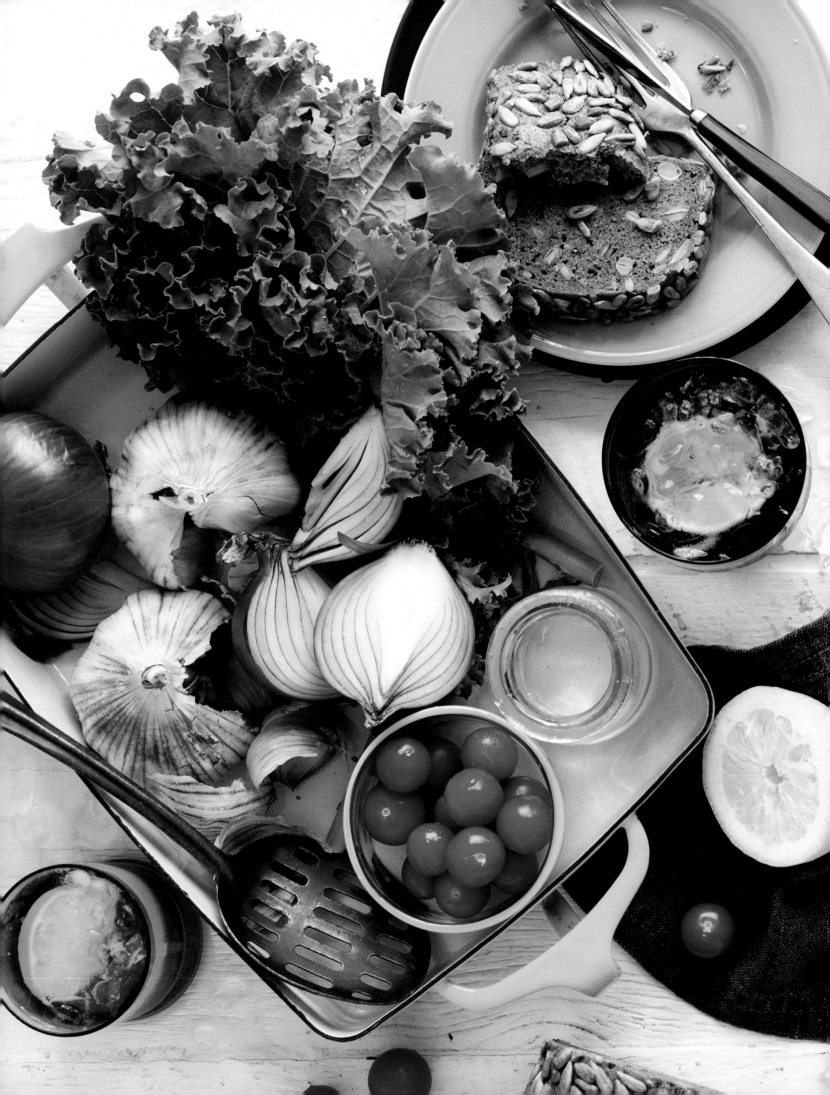

CONTENTS

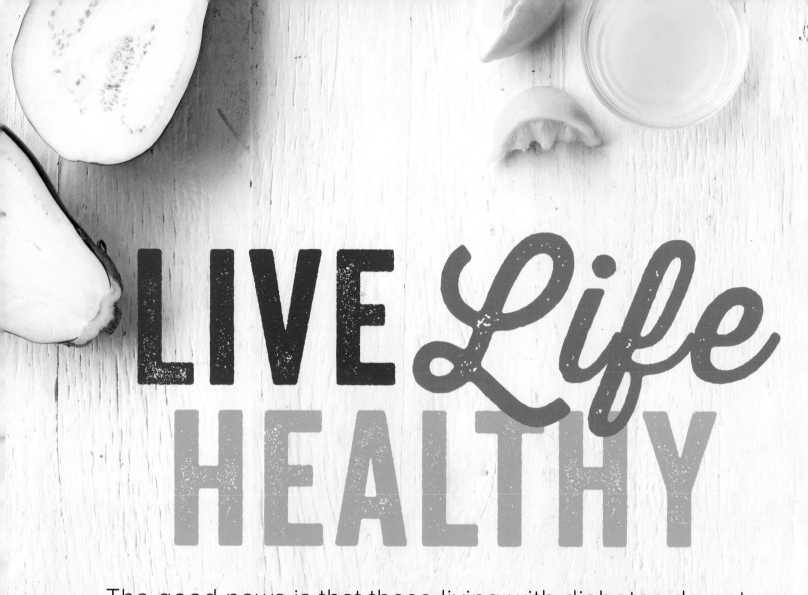

LIVE *Life* HEALTHY

The good news is that those living with diabetes do not need to follow a special diet, just the same healthy diet that is recommended for most of us. You don't need to buy special products or follow an extreme eating plan. However, what and how you eat does play an important role in managing the disease, so think of it as an added motivation to exercise and eat well.

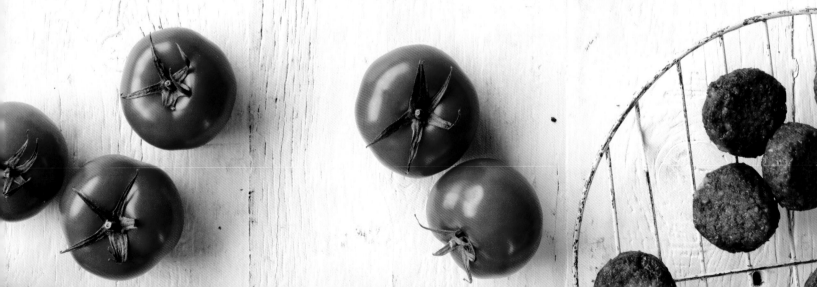

The key steps to managing diabetes

1 SIT LESS; MOVE MORE.

Activity and exercise help insulin to work more effectively in the body, and to get glucose into the muscle cells to be used to fuel the activity. The more time you spend sitting, the less fuel your body uses and the harder it is to control blood glucose levels. Aim for at least 30 minutes of exercise on most days. Walking is ideal. You can break this into two or three shorter walks if you prefer. In fact, a 10-15 minute walk after meals is a fantastic way to help get blood glucose back under control after eating.

2 KEEP A HEALTHY WEIGHT.

If you are overweight, losing even 5% of your body weight is enough to benefit your health and management of diabetes. So don't feel that you have failed if you don't reach your target weight. Following the healthy eating advice in this book, reducing portion sizes, ensuring you get enough sleep, regularly exercising and managing stress will help you reach and maintain a healthier weight.

3 EAT MORE PLANT FOOD.

A resounding message from nutrition research is that eating a plant-based diet is best for us all, whether or not you also eat meat. Plant food includes vegies, fruit, legumes (chickpeas, beans and lentils), wholegrains, nuts and seeds. Aim for at least 5-6 serves of different vegies and 2 serves of fruit each day.

4 CHOOSE GOOD FATS.

Gone are the days of the low-fat diet. It's now all about the right fats. Diets high in saturated fats are associated with increased insulin resistance and type 2 diabetes. Replacing saturated fat with primarily monounsaturated fats and some polyunsaturated fats can improve the action of insulin and lower your risk of cardiovascular disease. Aim to include more nuts, seeds, extra-virgin olive oil and avocado in your daily diet. Omega-3 fats in oily fish, such as sardines and tuna, are also terrific: aim for 2-3 serves a week.

5 CHOOSE SMART CARBS.

These are carbohydrate-containing foods that are digested slowly and therefore have far less impact on your blood glucose levels. They are nutrient-packed and often fibre-rich, so boost your health, and are associated with both a reduced risk of developing type 2 diabetes as well as helping with better diabetes management.

Smart carbs include whole fruit over fruit juice, reduced-fat milk and yoghurt, and minimally-processed wholegrains and legumes. At the same time, cut back on processed foods that contain refined starch and added sugars, such as soft drinks, lollies, biscuits, cakes, white bread (including bagels and crumpets), potatoes and white rice.

DISCLAIMER *The following information provides basic guidelines to healthy eating for people with diabetes. Please check with your doctor, dietitian or diabetes educator as to the suitability of this information for your diabetes management.*

14-DAY menu planner

DAY	BREAKFAST	SNACK	LUNCH	SNACK	DINNER	DESSERT	TOTAL DAILY INTAKE
MONDAY	strawberry and passionfruit breakfast trifle (page 12)	¼ cup unsalted mixed nuts	spinach and cheese snails (page 85)	1 small banana	spanish pork cutlets (page 133)	coffee granita (page 215)	45.8g total fat (9.2g saturated fat); 5410kJ (1292 cal); 129.7g carbohydrate; 89g protein; 45g fibre; 1027mg sodium
TUESDAY	chia and almond toasted muesli (page 19)	invigorating fruit and vegetable juice (page 59)	vietnamese pancakes with prawns (page 93)	1 small apple	miso broth with salmon and soba (page 145)	frozen peach lassi (page 211)	44.1g total fat (8.4g saturated fat); 6630kJ (1585 cal); 196.1g carbohydrate; 78.6g protein; 28.5g fibre; 1424mg sodium
WEDNESDAY	toast with avocado, tahini and sumac tomatoes (page 35)	½ cup blueberries with 1 small (100g) tub low-fat fruit yoghurt	spiced lentil and roasted kumara soup (page 66)	2 medium kiwi fruit	grilled steak with salsa verde and soft polenta (page 154)	passionfruit mousse (page 208)	48.7g total fat (8.9g saturated fat); 5436kJ (1299 cal); 118.2g carbohydrate; 77.2g protein; 33.1g fibre; 925mg sodium
THURSDAY	green smoothie (page 58)	avocado and trout with fennel tzatziki sandwich (page 122)	asian beef rolls (page 70)	1 small pear	indian-spiced patties with carrot raita (page 134)	strawberry and pomegranate baked custard tarts (page 216)	47.3g total fat (5g saturated fat); 6379kJ (1524 cal); 189.4g carbohydrate; 63.6g protein; 30.8g fibre; 1253mg sodium
FRIDAY	breakfast quesadillas (page 15)	orange berry smoothie (page 59)	roast pumpkin and zucchini risoni salad (page 89)	½ cup straw-berries	kitchari (page 157)	baked apples and raspberries with quinoa almond crumble (page 219)	47.1g total fat (9.1g saturated fat); 6325kJ (1510 cal); 201.5g carbohydrate; 50.4g protein; 37.7g fibre; 797mg sodium
SATURDAY	strawberry and ricotta pancakes with honey (page 23)	1 small banana	hot and sour prawn and chicken soup (page 77)	1 small apple	five-spice beef with wasabi sauce (page 137)	chocolate semifreddo (page 207)	37.4g total fat (10g saturated fat); 5878kJ (1767 cal); 164.4g carbohydrate; 91.5g protein; 24.1g fibre; 1186mg sodium
SUNDAY	grilled eggs with spiced fennel and spinach (page 16)	1 small (100g) tub low-fat fruit yoghurt	moroccan lamb and chickpea wraps (page 69)	1 small nectarine	sticky chicken with noodles (page 129)	spelt crêpes with rhubarb in rose syrup (page 200)	52.4g total fat (12.3g saturated fat); 5302kJ (1166 cal); 145.7g carbohydrate; 101.7g protein; 29.4g fibre; 1438mg sodium

14-DAY menu planner

DAY	BREAKFAST	SNACK	LUNCH	SNACK	DINNER	DESSERT	TOTAL DAILY INTAKE
MONDAY	roasted field mushrooms with garlic, spinach and ricotta (page 36)	1 small banana	ginger and chilli chicken rice paper rolls (page 114)	½ cup mixed berries with 1 small (100g) tub low-fat fruit yoghurt	lamb cutlets with smashed potatoes and brussels sprouts salad (page 166)	tropical jelly with coconut yoghurt (page 220)	39.4g total fat (11.6g saturated fat); 6473kJ (1546 cal); 158.1g carbohydrate; 113.7g protein; 37.7g fibre; 708mg sodium
TUESDAY	poached egg and avocado bruschetta (page 48)	½ cup fresh strawberries	chai roasted pumpkin soup with honey walnuts (page 121)	1 small pear	barbecued squid with lemon cracked wheat risotto (page 190)	nectarine and almond tarte tartin (page 228)	55.5g total fat (11g saturated fat); 5889kJ (14.6 cal); 151.9g carbohydrate; 58.1g protein; 34.6g fibre; 1243mg sodium
WEDNESDAY	berry semolina porridge (page 51)	1 apple plus 1 small (100g) tub low fat fruit yoghurt	mixed mushroom trencher with herb salad (page 118)	2 kiwi fruit	korean beef lettuce cups with pickled vegetables (page 161)	very berry ice-cream sandwiches (page 234)	42.8g total fat (9.4g saturated fat); 6997kJ (1672 cal); 209.5g carbohydrate; 92.9g protein; 35.4g fibre; 1203mg sodium
THURSDAY	grilled fruit salad with coconut yoghurt (page 44)	1 orange	lime and coriander beef salad (page 98)	1 small (100g) tub low-fat fruit yoghurt	kaffir lime and red curry fish parcels (page 169)	rhubarb and vanilla baked custard (page 227)	30g total fat (9.1g saturated fat); 5665kJ (1353 cal); 147.9g carbohydrate; 105.3g protein; 29.9g fibre; 1039mg sodium
FRIDAY	scrambled egg, smashed avocado and bean breakfast wrap (page 40)	1 apple	rocket, chicken and date salad (page 90)	½ cup blueberries	pork and sage meatballs with cabbage and pear (page 173)	roasted pears with cinnamon labne (page 224)	52.9g total fat (13.7g saturated fat); 6813kJ (1628 cal); 175.2g carbohydrate; 91.7g protein; 45.9g fibre; 741mg sodium
SATURDAY	pea fritters with avocado goat's cheese (page 52)	1 small banana	spiced vegetable, chickpea and ricotta salad (page 102)	2 kiwi fruit	salmon with green papaya and pink grapefruit salad (page 181)	orange and pomegranate steamed puddings (page 231)	73g total fat (18.2g saturated fat); 7519kJ (1796 cal); 183.4g carbohydrate; 82.8g protein; 37.2g fibre; 1265mg sodium
SUNDAY	baked bean and tomato pots with rosemary sourdough crumble (page 43)	1 pear	thai prawn burger (page 117)	½ cup strawberries with 1 small (100g) tub low-fat fruit yoghurt	baked chicken with maple parsnips (page 185)	caramel swirl ice-cream sandwiches (page 235)	44.3g total fat (8.1g saturated fat); 5796kJ (1385 cal); 150.2g carbohydrate; 81.5g protein; 42.4g fibre; 1288mg sodium

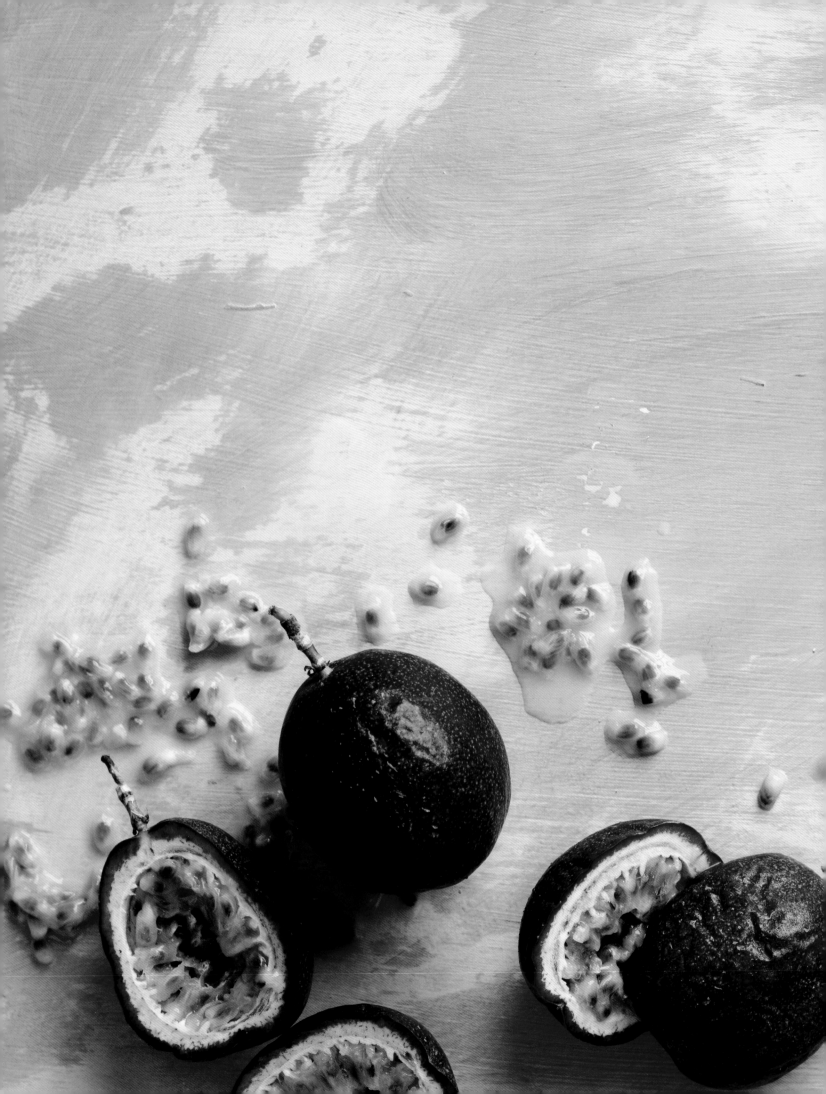

BREAKFAST

The most important meal of the day, breakfast helps restore and maintain control of blood sugar levels.

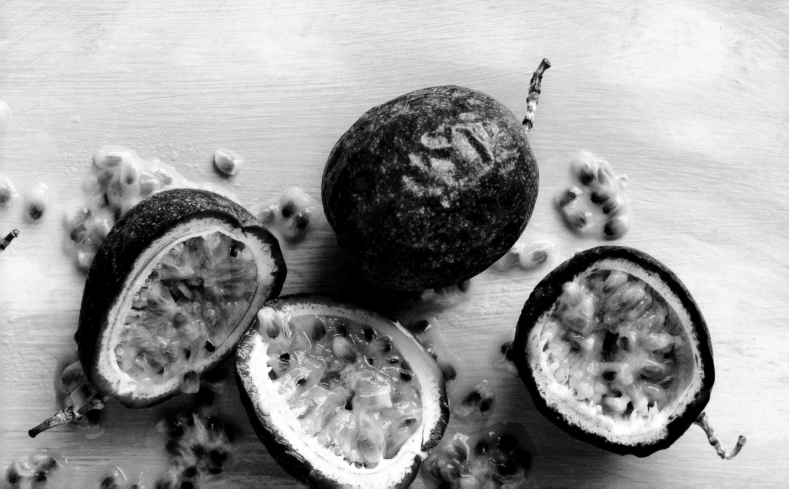

NUTRITIONAL COUNT PER SERVING

- 2g total fat
- 0.5g saturated fat
- 722kJ (172 cal)
- 36.1g carbohydrate
- 16.2g protein
- 15.5g fibre
- 411mg sodium
- low GI

strawberry & passionfruit breakfast trifle

PREP TIME 5 MINUTES ◆ SERVES 2

2 Weet-Bix (50g), broken into chunks

½ cup (40g) All-Bran cereal

⅓ cup (80ml) fresh passionfruit pulp

1 cup (280g) low-fat plain yoghurt

140g (1½ ounces) strawberries, sliced thinly

1 Layer half the Weet-Bix and All-Bran in two 1¼-cup (310ml) serving glasses. Top with half the passionfruit, yoghurt and strawberries.

2 Repeat with remaining Weet-Bix and All-Bran and yoghurt. Top with the remaining strawberries and drizzle with remaining passionfruit.

TIPS You will need about 4 passionfruit. You can make the trifle with any seasonal fruit combination or even with canned fruit in natural juices. Canned pears and frozen raspberries work well together.

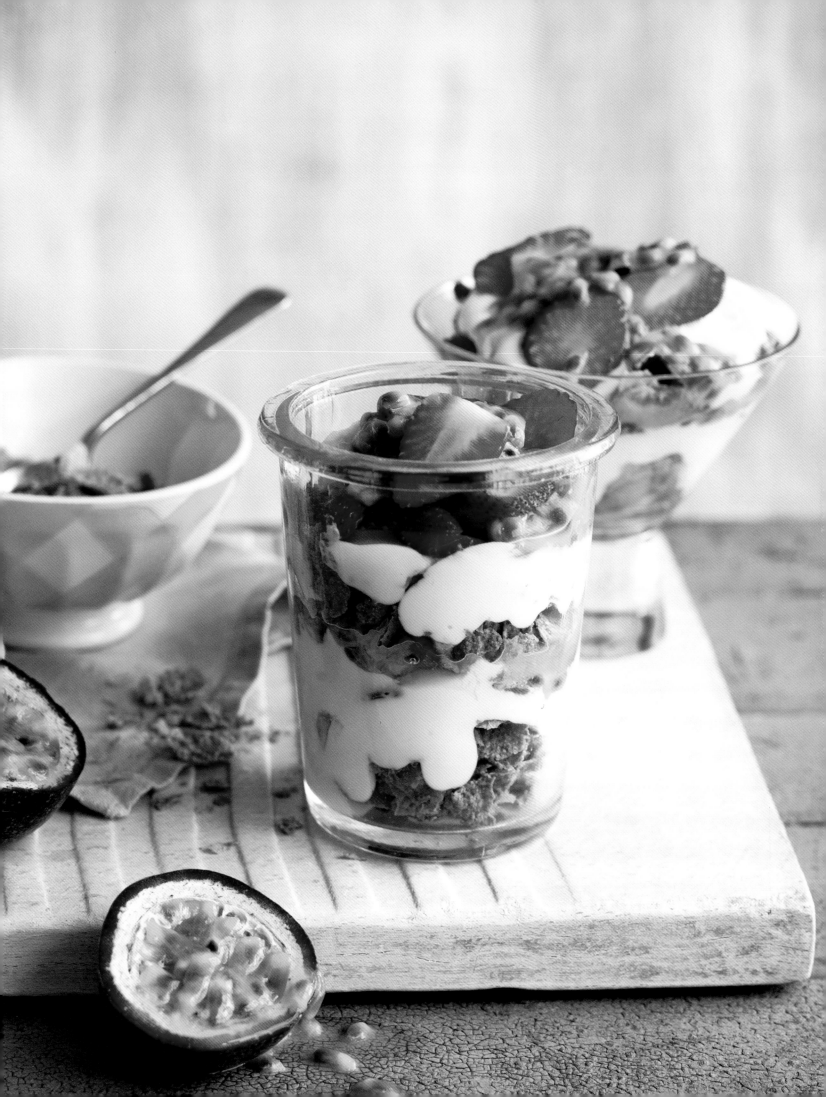

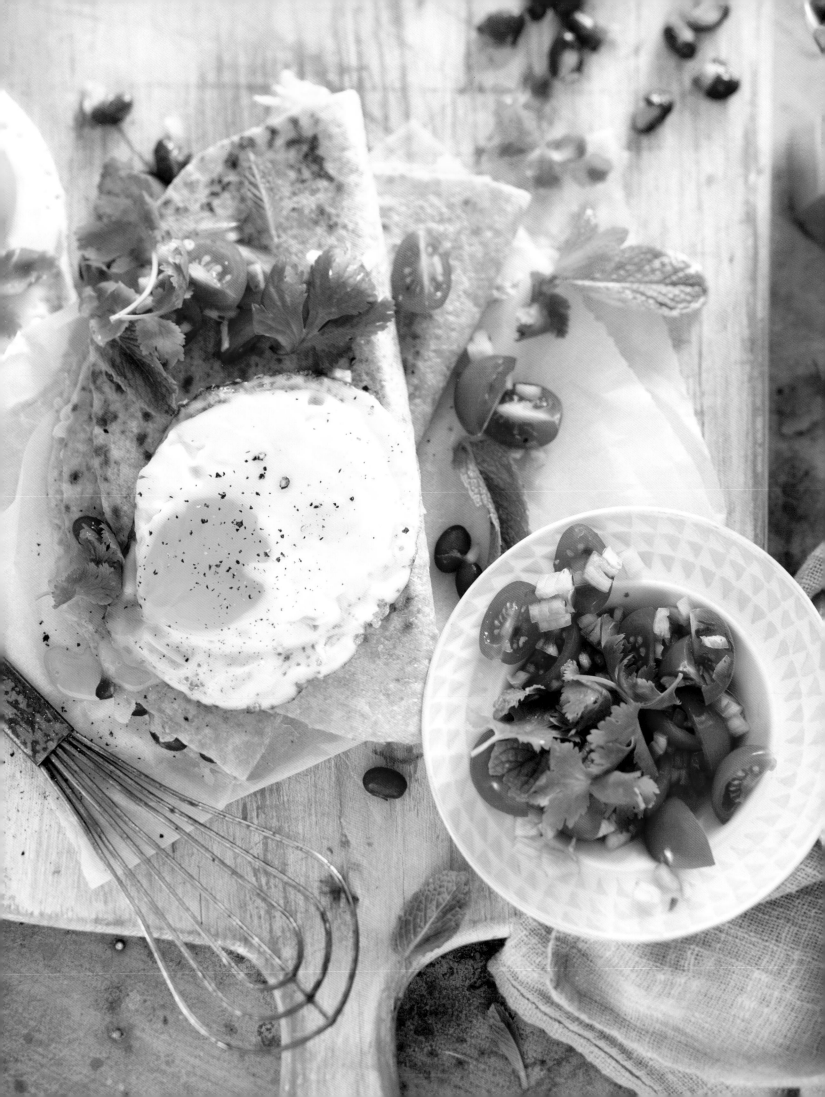

breakfast quesadillas

PREP + COOK TIME 20 MINUTES ◆ **SERVES** 2

125g (4 ounces) canned salt-reduced kidney beans, rinsed, drained, mashed

½ cup (85g) cooked brown rice

2 x 20cm (8-inch) wholemeal tortillas

⅓ cup (40g) grated extra-light tasty cheese

1 tablespoon olive oil

2 small eggs (100g)

TOMATO SALSA

160g (5 ounces) cherry tomatoes, chopped coarsely

2 tablespoons fresh coriander leaves (cilantro)

2 tablespoons fresh mint leaves

1 shallot (25g), chopped finely

2 teaspoons lemon juice

¼ teaspoon chilli flakes

1 Make tomato salsa.

2 Combine beans and rice in a medium bowl. Spoon the bean mixture over half of each tortilla and sprinkle with cheese. Fold over to enclose.

3 Heat half the oil in a large non-stick frying pan over medium heat; cook the quesadillas for 2 minutes each side or until brown and crisp. Set aside; cover to keep warm.

4 Heat remaining oil in same pan over low heat; cook eggs for 3 minutes or until cooked how you like them.

5 Top quesadillas with eggs and salsa.

TOMATO SALSA Combine ingredients in a medium bowl.

TIPS You can use microwave brown rice instead of cooking from raw, if you like. If you want to cook your own rice, cook ¼ cup of brown rice; use the ½ cup cooked rice required, and save the remainder for another use. You could also poach the eggs. Microwave tortillas in the packet to separate them if they are sticking together.

grilled eggs with spiced fennel and spinach

PREP + COOK TIME 20 MINUTES ◆ SERVES 2

2 teaspoons olive oil

1 clove garlic, crushed

1 fresh small red thai (serrano) chilli, sliced finely

½ small fennel bulb (100g), trimmed, sliced finely

100g (3 ounces) baby corn, halved

50g (1½ ounces) baby spinach leaves

2 eggs

1 tablespoon finely grated parmesan

2 slices rye sourdough bread (90g), toasted

1 Preheat grill (broiler) to high.

2 Heat oil in a large ovenproof non-stick frying pan over medium heat; cook garlic, chilli, fennel and corn, stirring occasionally, for 5 minutes or until fennel is soft. Add spinach; cook, stirring, for 1 minute or until spinach has wilted.

3 Make two holes in the spinach mixture; break one egg into each hole. Sprinkle with parmesan.

4 Place under grill for 2 minutes or until eggs are cooked as desired.

5 Serve eggs and spinach mixture with toast.

TIPS Reserve fennel fronds to sprinkle over eggs as a garnish. You need an ovenproof frying pan as it goes under the grill, or you can cover the pan handle with a few layers of foil to protect it from the heat.

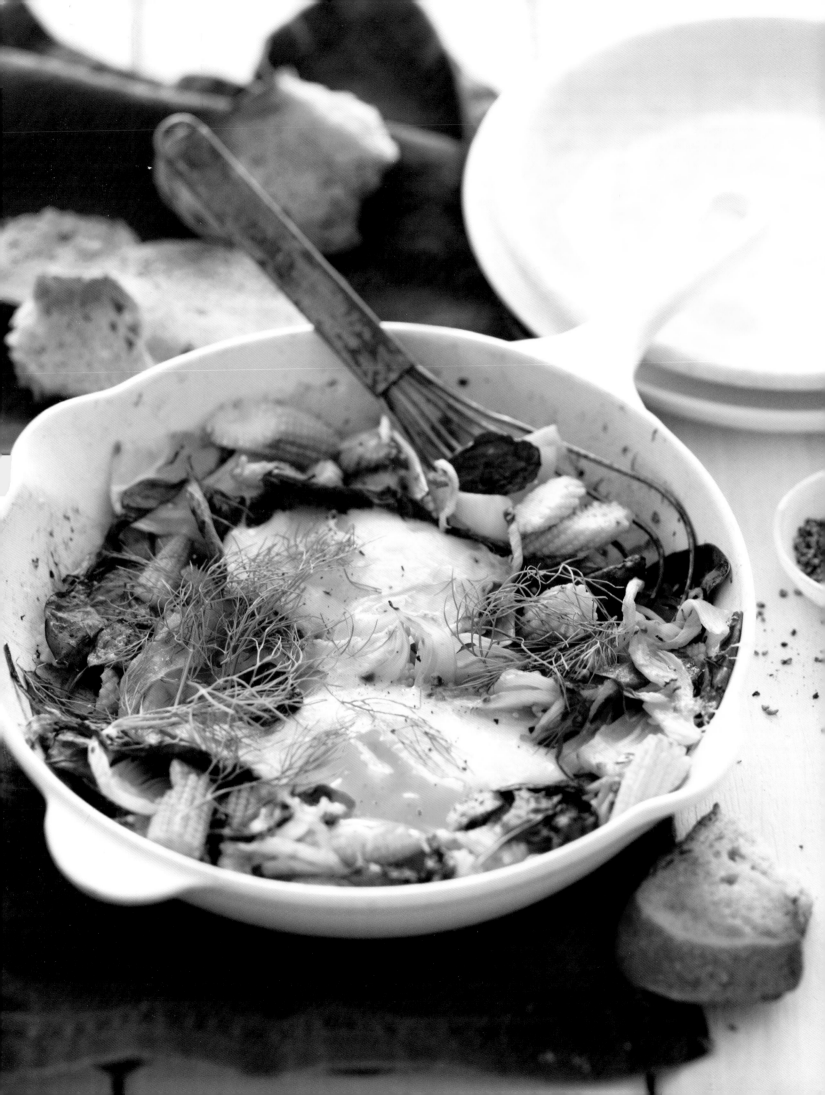

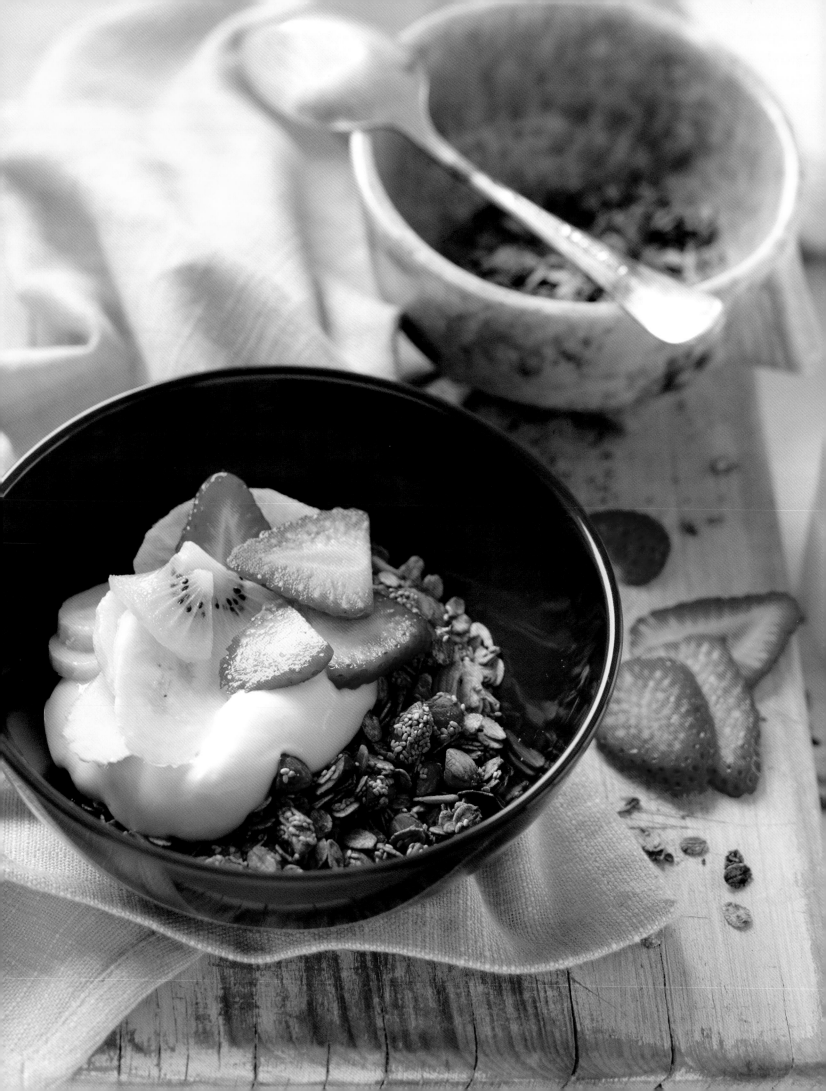

chia and almond toasted muesli

PREP + COOK TIME 20 MINUTES (+ COOLING) ◆ **SERVES** 2 (MAKES 1 CUP)

½ cup (45g) rolled oats

1 tablespoon chia seeds

2 tablespoons coarsely chopped almonds

¼ teaspoon mixed spice

2 teaspoons dark agave nectar

1 tablespoon sunflower seeds

1 tablespoon LSA

1 medium kiwi fruit (85g), sliced

50g (1½ ounces) strawberries, quartered

1 medium banana (200g), sliced

⅓ cup (95g) low-fat plain yoghurt

½ cup (125ml) skim milk

1 Preheat oven to 200°C/400°F.

2 Grease and line an oven tray with baking paper. Combine oats, chia, nuts and spice on tray. Drizzle with nectar; toss well. Bake for 10 minutes or until mixture is browned lightly. Cool on tray.

3 Transfer to a medium bowl; stir through seeds and LSA.

4 Divide evenly into two bowls. Top with fruit and yoghurt. Serve each with ¼ cup milk.

TIP Make double or triple the muesli recipe and store it in an airtight container in the fridge for up to 3 months.

omelette with asparagus and mint

PREP + COOK TIME 20 MINUTES ◆ MAKES 2

1 baby new potato (40g), cut into 5mm (¼-inch) cubes

170g (5½ ounces) asparagus, trimmed

1 cup (120g) frozen peas

2 eggs

⅓ cup coarsely chopped fresh mint leaves

1 tablespoon olive oil

2 slices rye sourdough bread (90g), toasted

1 Cook potato in a small saucepan of boiling water for 3 minutes; add asparagus and peas, cook a further 1 minute or until asparagus is bright green and potato is tender; drain. When cool enough to handle, cut the asparagus in half; finely slice the stem ends crossways.

2 Lightly whisk eggs in a medium bowl; stir in potato, peas, mint and chopped asparagus ends.

3 Heat half the oil in a small non-stick frying pan on high; cook half the egg mixture for about 2 minutes, pulling in the egg with a spatula to help it cook quickly. Fold over; slide onto a warm serving plate. Repeat with remaining oil and egg mixture to make second omelette.

4 Top omelettes with remaining asparagus and serve with toast.

TIPS If you are pressed for time, make one big omelette in a medium frying pan. You can change the filling depending on the seasonal vegetables available – try adding pumpkin or broccolini.

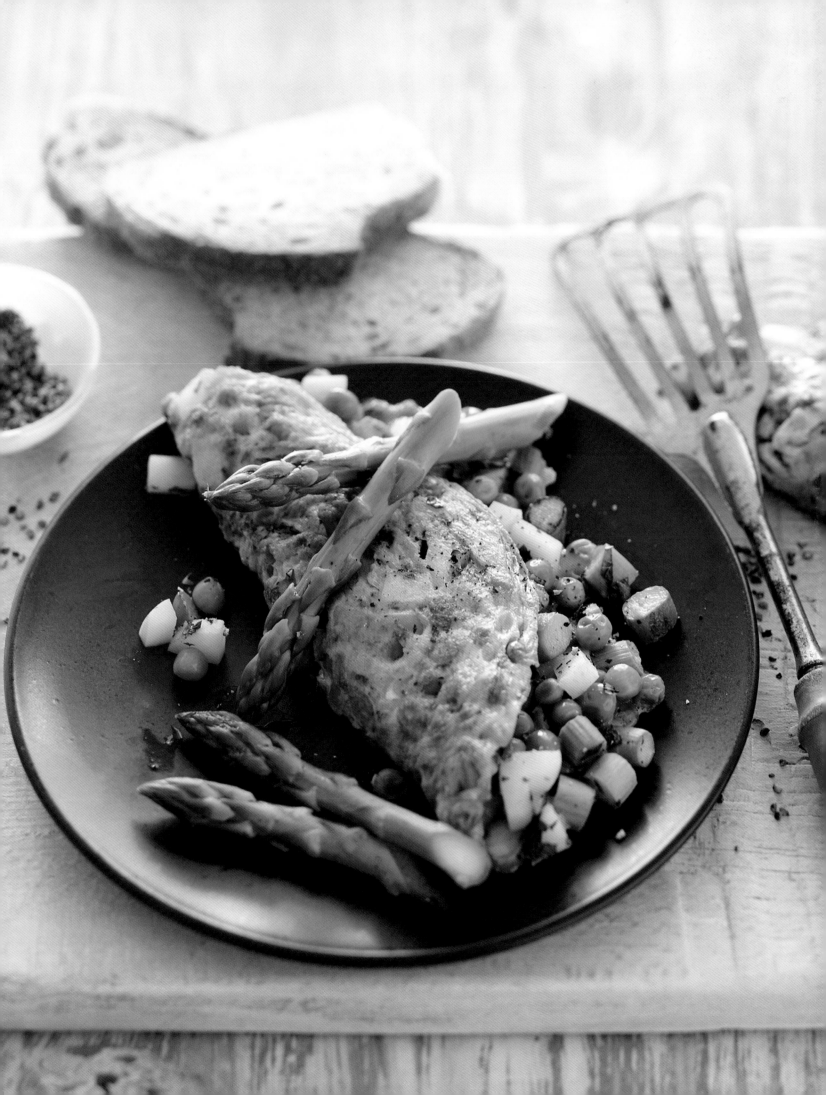

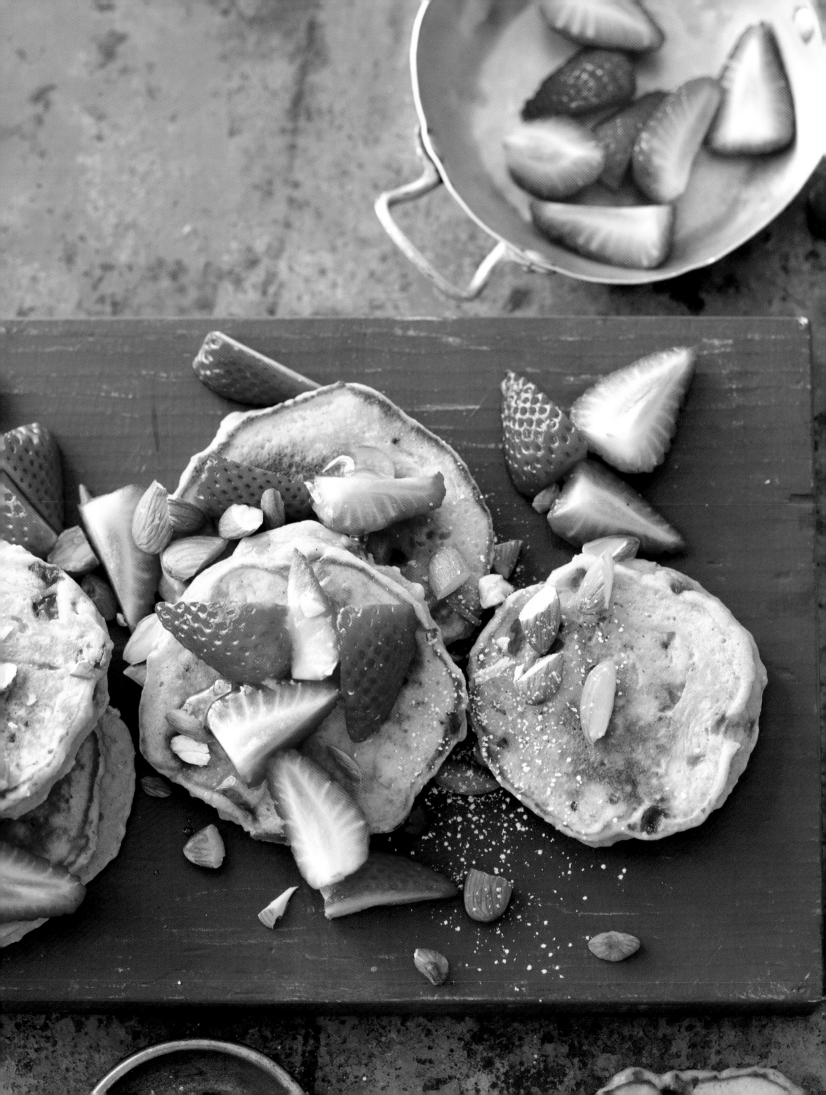

NUTRITIONAL COUNT PER SERVING

● 14.5g total fat   ● 16.2g protein
● 4.2g saturated fat   ● 5.7g fibre
● 1812kJ (433 cal)   ● 291mg sodium
● 57.5g carbohydrate   ● low GI

strawberry and ricotta pancakes with honey

PREP + COOK TIME 20 MINUTES ◆ SERVES 2

⅓ cup (80g) low-fat ricotta

2 eggs, separated

2 tablespoons caster (superfine) sugar

1 teaspoon vanilla extract

¼ cup (35g) buckwheat flour

⅓ cup (50g) wholemeal self-raising flour

¼ cup (45g) finely chopped strawberries

cooking-oil spray

150g (4½ ounces) strawberries, quartered

1 tablespoon coarsely chopped almonds

2 teaspoons honey

1 Whisk ricotta, egg yolks, sugar and extract in a small bowl. Stir in sifted flours and finely chopped strawberries.

2 Beat egg whites in a small bowl with an electric mixer until soft peaks form. Fold through ricotta mixture in two batches.

3 Spray a medium frying pan with oil; heat over medium heat. Spoon ¼ cup of batter into pan; cook pancakes for 3 minutes each side or until golden. Repeat with remaining batter.

4 Serve pancakes with extra strawberries and nuts; drizzle with honey.

serving suggestion Dust each serve with ¼ teaspoon icing (confectioners') sugar, if you like.

TIPS You can slightly spread the pancakes with the back of a spoon if the mixture doesn't spread when you add it to the pan. These pancakes are also great for dessert. You can make little pancakes, if you prefer, using just 1 tablespoon of mixture. Swap the strawberries for bananas, if you like.

fatteh

PREP + COOK TIME 15 MINUTES ◆ SERVES 2

420g (12½ ounces) canned
no-added-salt chickpeas
(garbanzo beans), rinsed, drained

⅓ cup (80ml) water

1 wholemeal lebanese bread (80g)

3 teaspoons olive oil

1½ cups (420g) low-fat plain yoghurt

1 clove garlic, crushed

¼ cup (40g) pine nuts, toasted

¼ teaspoon sumac

This is a typical Lebanese breakfast dish. It's usually served on a big plate so friends, family, and even the neighbours, can share.

1 Combine chickpeas and the water in a small saucepan over medium heat. Bring to the boil, reduce heat to low; simmer, covered, for 5 minutes. Using a potato masher, roughly mash chickpeas; keep warm.

2 Preheat grill (broiler) to medium. Brush bread with oil; place on an oven tray. Grill both sides until bread is dry and crisp (be careful not to burn the bread). Break bread into pieces.

3 Combine yoghurt and garlic in a small bowl.

4 To serve, divide bread pieces between two shallow plates; spoon over warm chickpea mash. Top with yoghurt mixture; scatter with pine nuts and sprinkle with sumac. Serve immediately.

TIPS If you find the chickpea mixture too thick, add an extra teaspoon or two of hot water. You can easily double the recipe for a brunch with friends. If you prefer, crisp the bread in a 200°C/400°F oven for about 5 minutes.

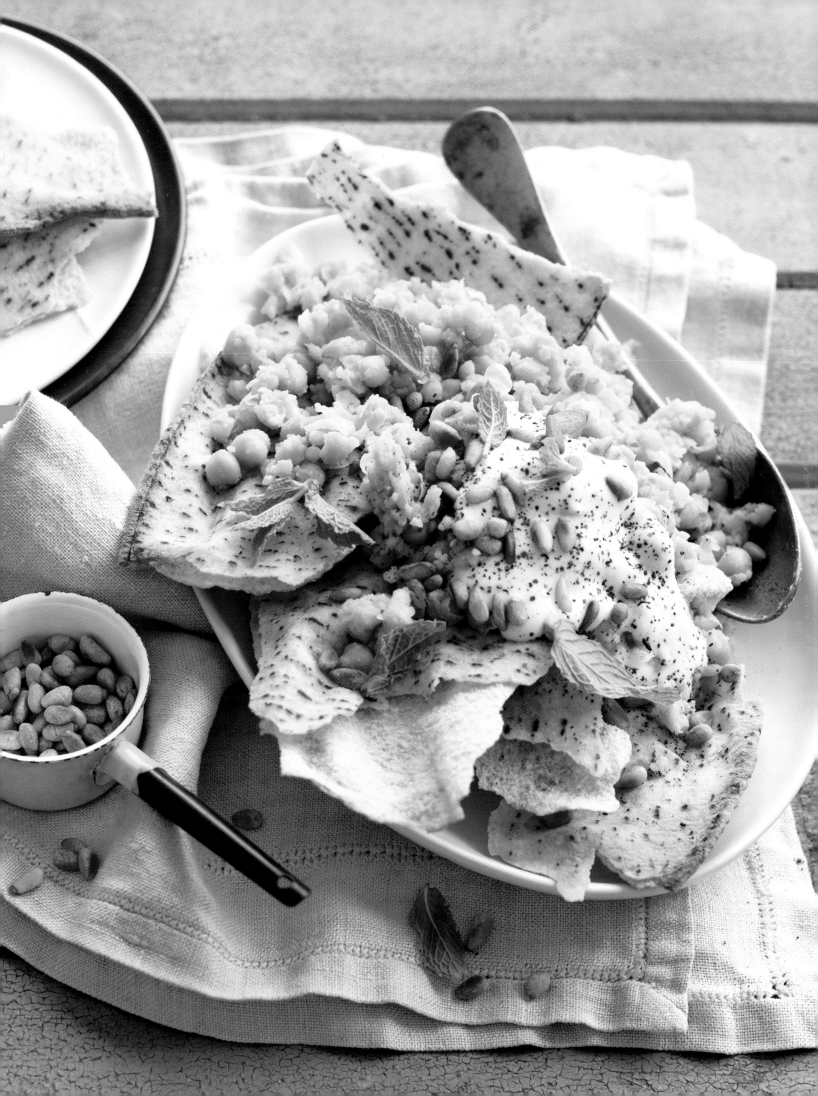

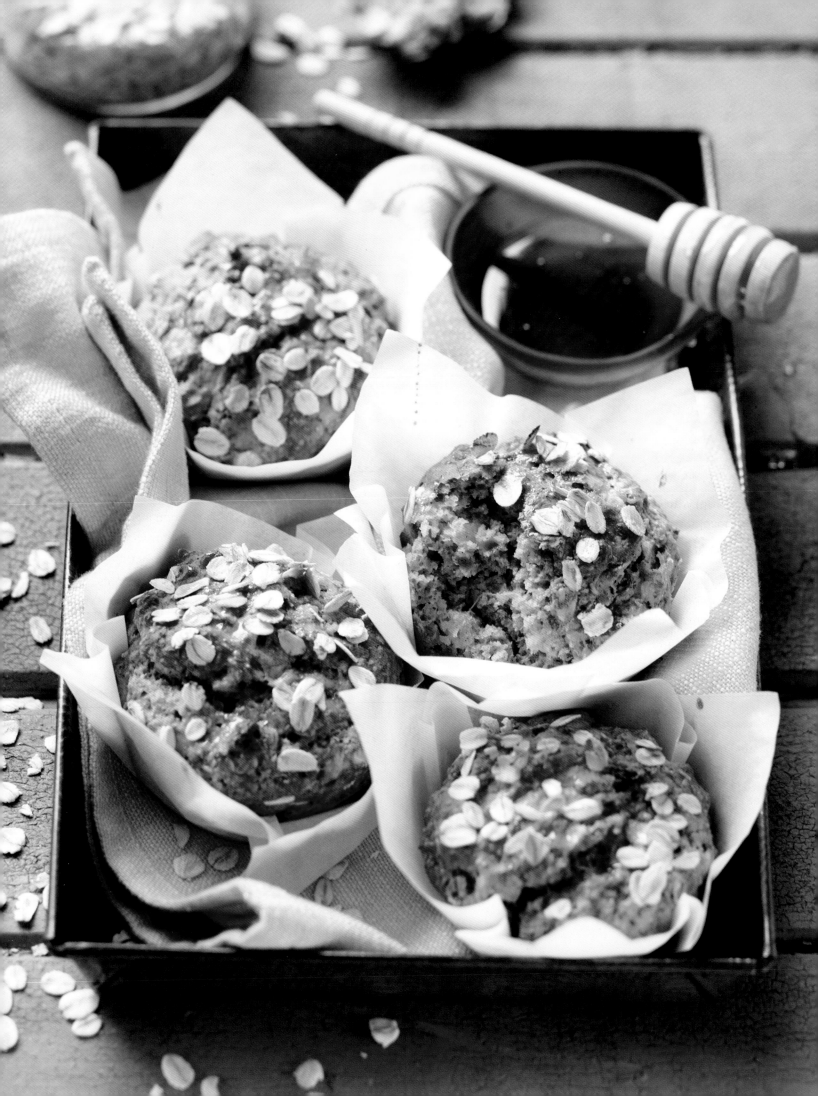

breakfast muffins

PREP + COOK TIME 40 MINUTES ◆ **MAKES** 4

¼ cup (20g) rolled oats

¾ cup (120g) wholemeal plain (all-purpose) flour

1 teaspoon ground cinnamon

½ teaspoon baking powder

¼ teaspoon bicarbonate of soda (baking soda)

2 tablespoons sultanas

1 egg, beaten lightly

¼ cup (60ml) buttermilk

¼ cup (55g) apple puree

¼ cup (75g) mashed banana

1 teaspoon vanilla extract

1 teaspoon honey, warmed

1 Preheat oven to 200°C/400°F. Line four holes of a 6-hole (¾-cup/180ml) texas muffin pan with baking paper squares or muffin cases.

2 Reserve 2 teaspoons of the oats. Sift flour, cinnamon, baking powder and soda in a medium bowl. Add sultanas and the remaining oats to the flour mixture; stir in combined egg, buttermilk, puree, banana and extract.

3 Divide mixture among prepared pan holes; sprinkle with reserved oats. Bake for 20 minutes.

4 Brush tops with honey. Bake a further 5 minutes or until golden and cooked when tested with a skewer. Stand muffins in pan for 5 minutes before turning, top-side up, onto a wire rack to cool.

TIPS You need 1 small ripe banana (130g), to get the amount of mashed banana needed for these muffins. Muffins are suitable to freeze, stored in an airtight container, for up to 3 months. The muffins are best eaten warm; reheat, one at a time, in a microwave oven for about 20 seconds on HIGH (100%).

soy porridge with banana, whole seeds and almonds

PREP + COOK TIME 10 MINUTES ◆ SERVES 2

1 cup (90g) rolled oats

1½ cups (375ml) reduced-fat soy milk

¼ teaspoon ground cinnamon

1 tablespoon coarsely chopped dry-roasted almonds

¼ teaspoon each poppy seeds, sesame seeds, black chia seeds and linseeds

2 teaspoons sunflower seeds

½ medium banana (165g), sliced thickly

2 teaspoons pure maple syrup

1 Place oats, soy milk and cinnamon in a small saucepan over low heat, bring to a gentle simmer; cook, stirring occasionally, for 5 minutes or until mixture has thickened and oats are tender.

2 Meanwhile, combine nuts and seeds in a small bowl.

3 Serve porridge topped with banana; sprinkle with nut and seed mixture, drizzle with maple syrup.

TIPS Use traditional rolled oats rather than instant oats for a better texture. You can use white chia seeds, if you like. Swap banana for a low-GI fruit such as strawberries, grapes, peaches or plums.

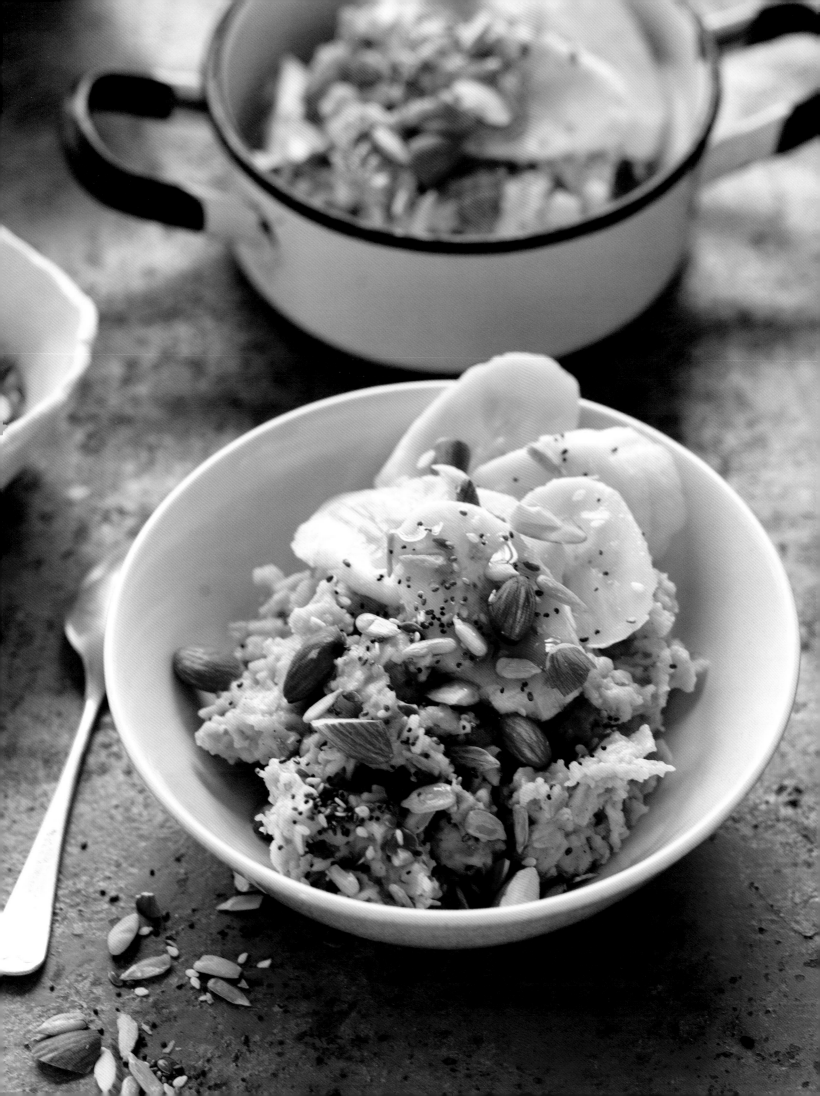

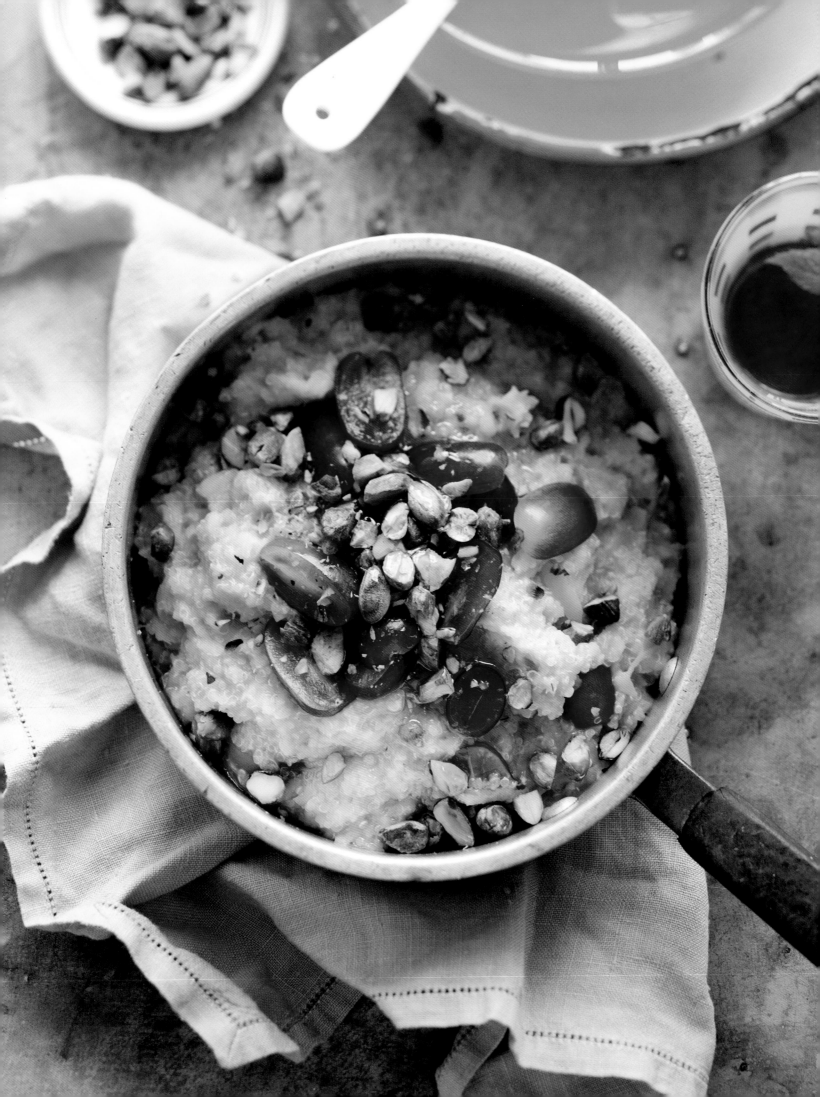

NUTRITIONAL COUNT PER SERVING

● 8.9g total fat   ● 12.2g protein

● 1g saturated fat   ● 5.6g fibre

● 1642kJ (392 cal)   ● 53mg sodium

● 63g carbohydrate   ● low GI

quinoa porridge

PREP + COOK TIME 20 MINUTES ◆ SERVES 2

½ cup (100g) white quinoa, rinsed, drained

1½ cups (375ml) water

½ cup (125ml) skim milk

1 medium apple (150g), grated coarsely

100g (3 ounces) red seedless grapes, halved

2 tablespoons pistachios, toasted, chopped coarsely

1 tablespoon honey

1 Combine quinoa and the water in a small saucepan; bring to the boil. Reduce heat; simmer, covered, for 10 minutes. Add milk; cook, covered, for a further 5 minutes or until quinoa is tender.

2 Stir in apple and half the grapes.

3 Serve porridge, topped with remaining grapes, nuts and drizzled with honey.

TIPS We used a pink lady apple in this recipe. Most quinoa comes rinsed, but it's a good habit to rinse it yourself under cold water until the water runs clear, then drain it. This removes any remaining outer coating, which has a bitter taste. Quinoa absorbs a lot of liquid. Depending how you like your porridge, add a little boiling water at the end of step 1 to thin it out.

zucchini and corn frittatas

PREP + COOK TIME 40 MINUTES ◆ SERVES 2

3 teaspoons semolina

2 small zucchini (180g)

1 baby new potato (40g), unpeeled

2 eggs

⅓ cup (80g) low-fat ricotta

1 tablespoon creamed corn

1 tablespoon finely chopped fresh flat-leaf parsley

150g (4½ ounces) truss cherry tomatoes

2 teaspoons olive oil

2 slices soy linseed sourdough bread (90g), toasted

1 Preheat oven to 220°C/425°F. Lightly grease two holes of a 6-hole (¾-cup/180ml) texas muffin pan. Sprinkle greased holes with semolina.

2 Using a vegetable peeler; cut one zucchini into ribbons. Line pan holes with zucchini, overlapping at slightly different angles. Coarsely grate remaining zucchini and potato, squeezing out excess liquid.

3 Whisk eggs, ricotta, corn, parsley, grated zucchini and potato in a small bowl. Spoon into prepared holes. Bake for 25 minutes.

4 Place tomatoes on an oven tray; drizzle with oil. Bake for 10 minutes with frittatas until tomatoes soften and frittatas are golden and set.

5 Serve frittatas and tomatoes; accompany with toast.

TIP These frittatas are great to pack for a work lunch as they can be eaten warm or cold. Make them a day ahead and reheat in a microwave oven on MEDIUM (50%) for about 2 minutes or until heated through.

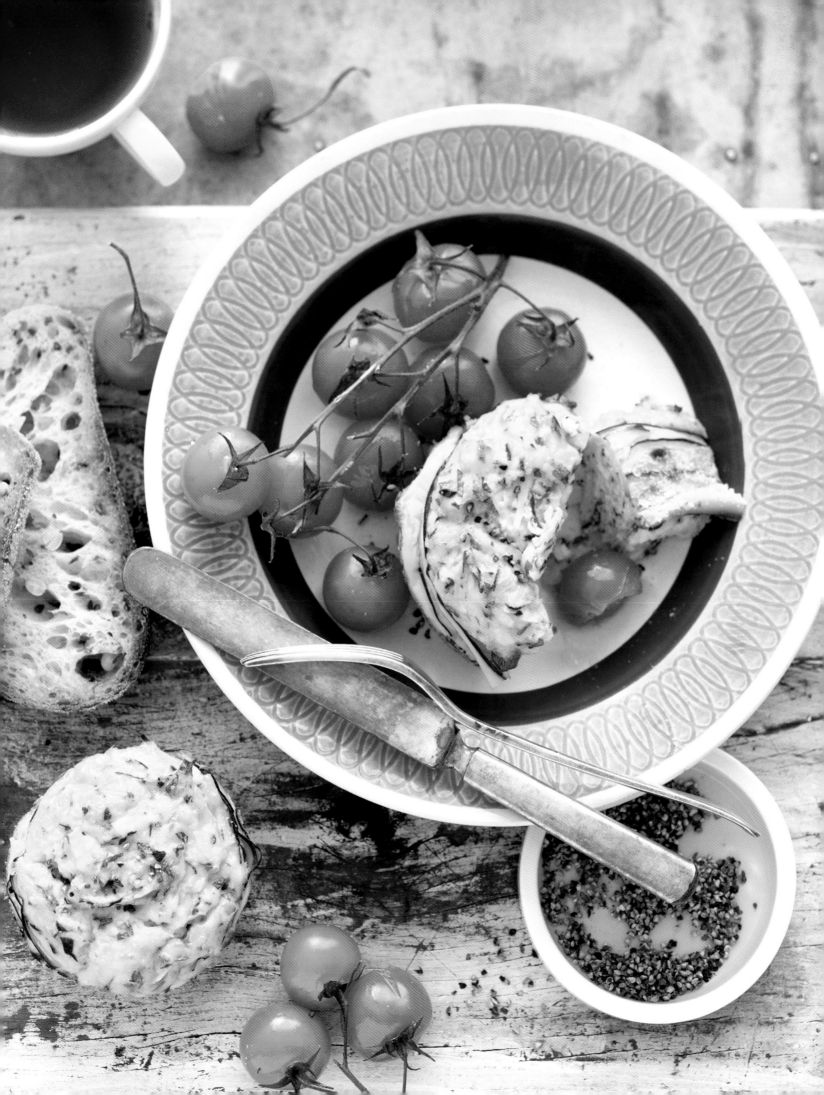

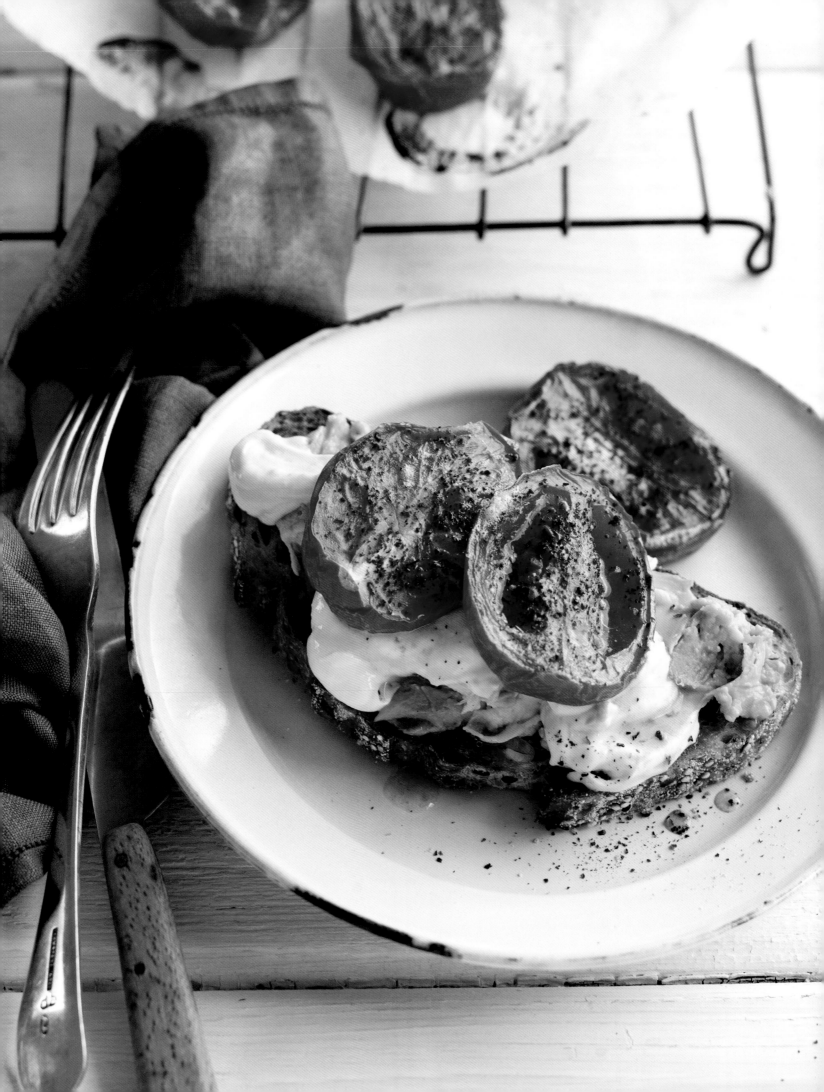

NUTRITIONAL COUNT PER SERVING

● 17.4g total fat   ● 12.2g protein
● 3g saturated fat   ● 7.2g fibre
● 1490kJ (356 cal)   ● 371mg sodium
● 33.5g carbohydrate   ● low GI

toast with avocado, tahini and sumac tomatoes

PREP + COOK TIME 40 MINUTES ◆ SERVES 2

3 medium roma (egg) tomatoes (225g), halved lengthways

½ teaspoon sumac

cooking-oil spray

½ clove garlic, crushed

¼ cup (70g) low-fat plain yoghurt

1 tablespoon tahini (sesame seed paste)

1 teaspoon lemon juice

½ small avocado (100g)

2 slices wholegrain sourdough bread (120g), toasted

1 Preheat oven to 180°C/350°F.

2 Grease and line a small oven tray with baking paper. Place tomato on tray, skin-side down; sprinkle sumac over cut surfaces, spray lightly with olive oil. Roast for 30 minutes or until tomato has collapsed slightly.

3 Place garlic, yoghurt, tahini and juice in a small bowl; whisk to combine.

4 Spread half the avocado thickly over each toast slice. Spoon tahini mixture over avocado and top with tomatoes.

TIPS We cut the sourdough into 1.5cm (3/4-inch) slices. Cook extra sumac tomatoes and keep them in the fridge to have on hand and use as a delicious ingredient in pasta, salads and sandwiches. Store them in an airtight container for up to a week.

roasted field mushrooms with garlic, spinach and ricotta

PREP + COOK TIME 40 MINUTES ◆ SERVES 2

4 medium portobello field mushrooms (400g), trimmed

275g (9 ounces) baby truss tomatoes

rice bran oil spray

2 cloves garlic, crushed

1 tablespoon balsamic vinegar

1 teaspoon extra virgin olive oil

12 sprigs fresh thyme

50g (1½ ounces) baby spinach leaves

¼ cup (25g) low-fat ricotta cheese

3 slices multigrain bread (135g), toasted

1 Preheat oven to 200°C/400°F. Line a large baking dish with baking paper.

2 Place mushrooms and tomato in baking dish. Spray lightly with oil. Season with pepper.

3 Combine garlic, vinegar and olive oil in a small bowl; drizzle over mushrooms, sprinkle mushrooms with thyme. Cover pan loosely with baking paper. Bake for 20 minutes.

4 Discard top baking paper. Tuck spinach leaves under mushrooms and tomato. Dollop mushrooms with ricotta. Bake, uncovered, for 5 minutes or until vegetables are tender. Serve with toast.

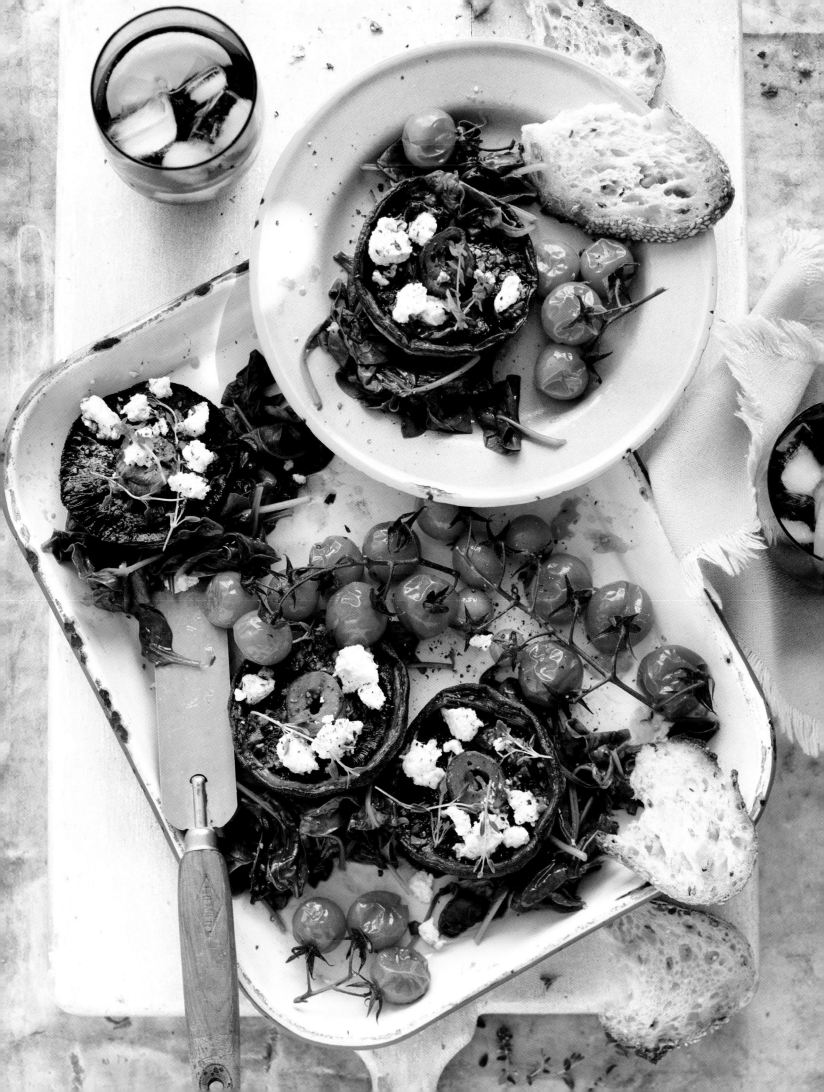

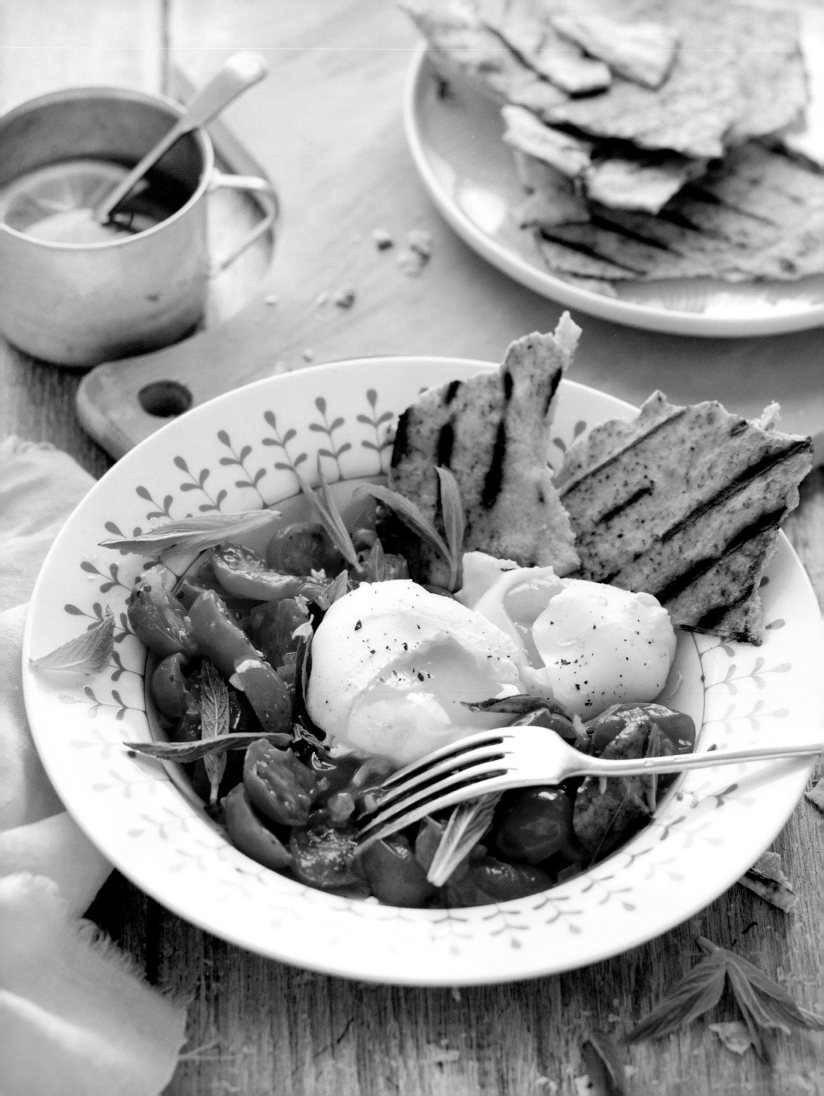

indian-style tomatoes and eggs

PREP + COOK TIME 45 MINUTES ◆ **SERVES** 2

2 teaspoons rice bran oil

1 small brown onion (80g), chopped finely

1 long fresh red chilli, seeded, chopped finely

2 cloves garlic, crushed

½ teaspoon each brown mustard seeds and cumin seeds

2 tablespoons fresh curry leaves

400g (12½ ounces) grape tomatoes, halved

4 small eggs

1 wholemeal lebanese bread (80g)

¼ cup firmly packed fresh mint leaves

1 Heat oil in a large non-stick pan over medium-low heat; cook onion and chilli, covered, for 5 minutes, stirring occasionally, or until onion is soft. Add garlic, seeds and curry leaves; cook, stirring, for 1 minute or until fragrant. Add tomato; cook, stirring, for 5 minutes or until softened. Season with pepper.

2 Meanwhile, half fill a large shallow frying pan with water; bring to the boil. Break 1 egg into a cup then slide into pan; repeat with remaining eggs. When all eggs are in the pan, allow water to return to the boil. Cover pan, turn off heat; stand for 3 minutes or until a light film of egg white sets over yolks.

3 Using a slotted spoon remove eggs, one at a time, from pan; drain on kitchen paper, cover to keep warm.

4 Heat a grill pan (or grill or barbecue) over high heat; cook bread for 1 minute each side or until lightly charred. Cut toast into wedges.

5 Divide tomato mixture between plates; top with eggs, sprinkle with mint. Serve with toast.

TIP If fresh curry leaves aren't available use dried leaves.

scrambled eggs, smashed avocado and bean breakfast wrap

PREP + COOK TIME 20 MINUTES ◆ SERVES 2

1 small avocado (100g)

2 teaspoons lime juice

2 teaspoons finely grated lime rind

130g (4 ounces) rinsed, drained canned kidney beans

1 medium tomato (150g), chopped finely

½ small red onion (50g), sliced thinly

1 long fresh green chilli, sliced thinly

¼ cup loosely packed fresh coriander leaves (cilantro)

2 eggs

2 egg whites

1 tablespoon skim milk

1 tablespoon coarsely chopped fresh coriander (cilantro) leaves

1 teaspoon rice bran oil

4 rye mountain bread wraps (100g)

1   Mash avocado, juice and half the rind roughly in a small bowl with a fork. Season with pepper.

2   Combine kidney beans, tomato, onion, chilli, coriander leaves and remaining rind in a small bowl. Season with black pepper.

3   Whisk eggs, egg whites, milk and chopped coriander in a small bowl until combined.

4   Heat oil in a medium non-stick frying pan over medium-low heat; cook egg mixture, stirring gently, for 2 minutes or until just set.

5   Place two wraps together. Spread wrap with half the avocado mixture; top with half the bean mixture and half the scrambled egg. Roll up to form a wrap; cut in half. Repeat with remaining wraps.

TIPS We used two mountain bread wraps for each serve, this helps the wrap stay together as one wrap tends to be fragile. We used 1/2 x 400g (12 1/2 ounce) can salt-reduced kidney beans for this recipe. Omit the chilli or remove the seeds, if you like.

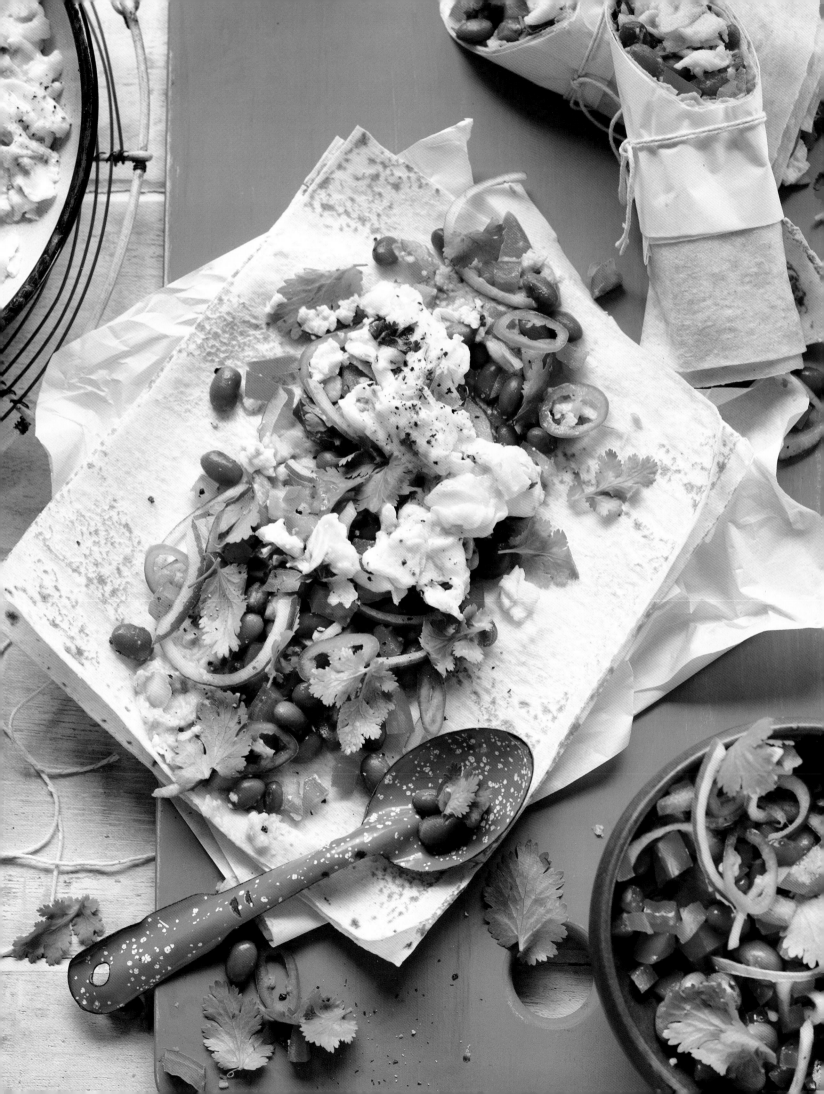

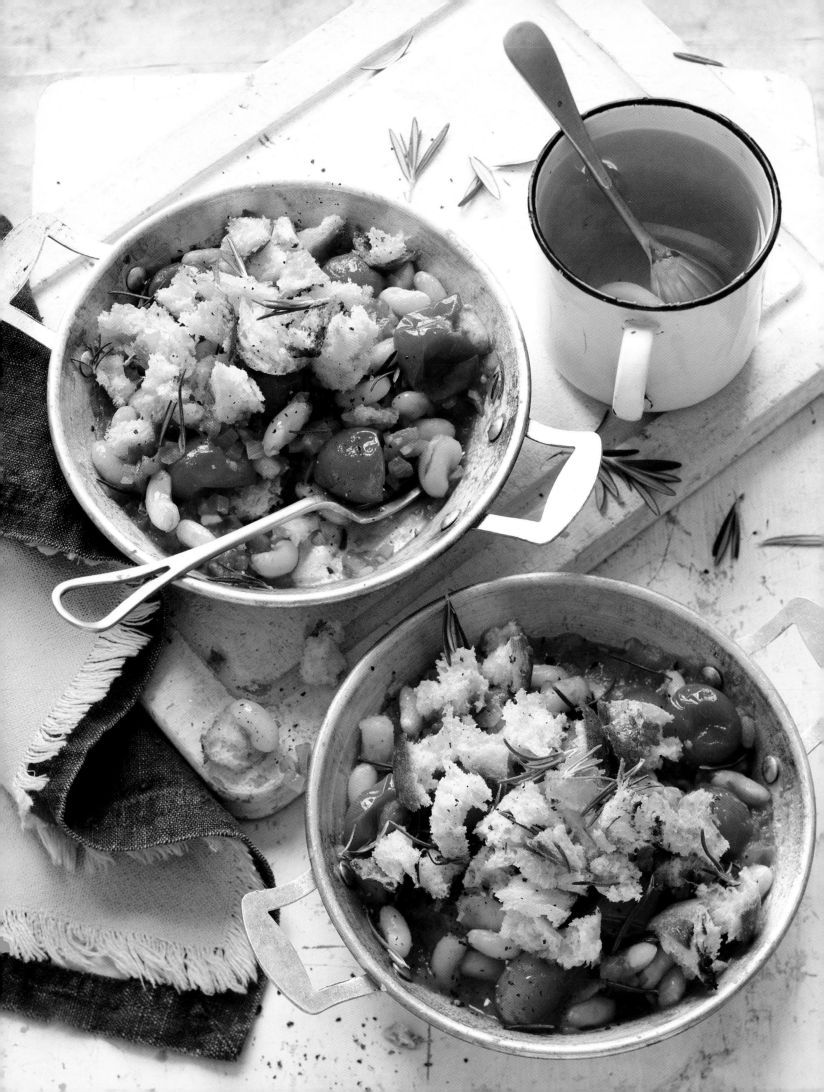

NUTRITIONAL COUNT PER SERVING

● 13.1g total fat ● 21.5g protein
● 1.9g saturated fat ● 16.1g fibre
● 1459kJ (349 cal) ● 310mg sodium
● 30.3g carbohydrate ● low GI

baked beans and tomato pots with rosemary sourdough crumble

PREP + COOK TIME 2½ HOURS (+ STANDING) ◆ **SERVES** 2

½ cup (100g) dried cannellini beans

rice bran oil spray

1 medium brown onion (150g), chopped finely

2 cloves garlic, crushed

1½ teaspoons chopped fresh rosemary

1 teaspoon ground cumin

pinch chilli flakes

400g (12½ ounces) canned cherry tomatoes in juice

1 cup (250ml) water

60g (2 ounces) white sourdough bread, torn roughly

1 tablespoon small fresh rosemary sprigs

Start this recipe the day before.

1 Cover beans in a large bowl with cold water; stand 8 hours or overnight. Drain.

2 Cook beans in a large saucepan of boiling water for 45 minutes or until tender. Drain.

3 Preheat oven to 200°C/400°F.

4 Spray a medium non-stick frying pan with oil, heat over low heat; cook onion, stirring, for 10 minutes or until softened. Add garlic, rosemary, cumin and chilli; cook, stirring, for 1 minute or until fragrant. Add tomatoes, the water and beans, bring to the boil; reduce heat, simmer, uncovered, for 10 minutes or until thickened slightly. Season with pepper.

5 Spoon mixture into 2 x 1½-cup (375ml) ovenproof dishes; place on a baking tray. Top mixture with torn bread and rosemary sprigs. Spray with oil.

6 Bake for 15 minutes or until browned and bubbling.

TIP You can use canned cannellini beans, but be aware that the sodium content of your meal will increase.

NUTRITIONAL COUNT PER SERVING

- 4g total fat
- 2.1g saturated fat
- 953kJ (228 cal)
- 36.8g carbohydrate
- 5.6g protein
- 10g fibre
- 37mg sodium
- low GI

grilled fruit salad with coconut yoghurt

PREP + COOK TIME 15 MINUTES ◆ **SERVES** 2

1 medium pear (230g), cored, cut into eight wedges

4 medium figs (240g), halved lengthways

1 medium blood orange (240g), peeled, cut into 1cm (½-inch) thick slices

⅓ cup (95g) coconut yoghurt

3 teaspoons sunflower seeds, toasted

1 Cook pear on a heated lightly oiled grill plate (or grill or barbecue), over medium-high heat, for 4 minutes each side or until slightly tender and charred.

2 Add figs halfway through cooking time; cook for 2 minutes each side until figs are tender and charred.

3 Combine grilled fruit with orange in serving bowls; top with yoghurt and sunflower seeds.

TIPS To cook figs, place a small sheet of baking paper on the grill plate to prevent the figs from sticking. You could also eat this fruit salad fresh without grilling the fruit, for a breakfast on-the-go. Pure coconut yoghurt is dairy-free and is available from health food stores.

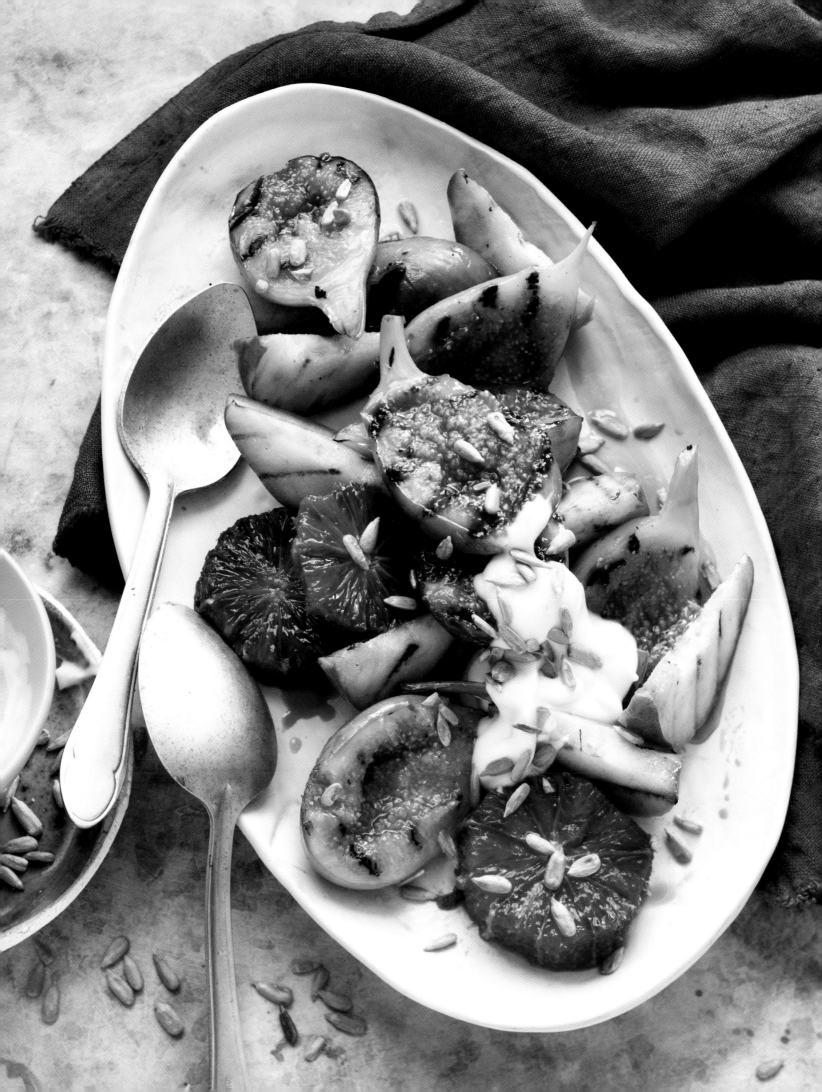

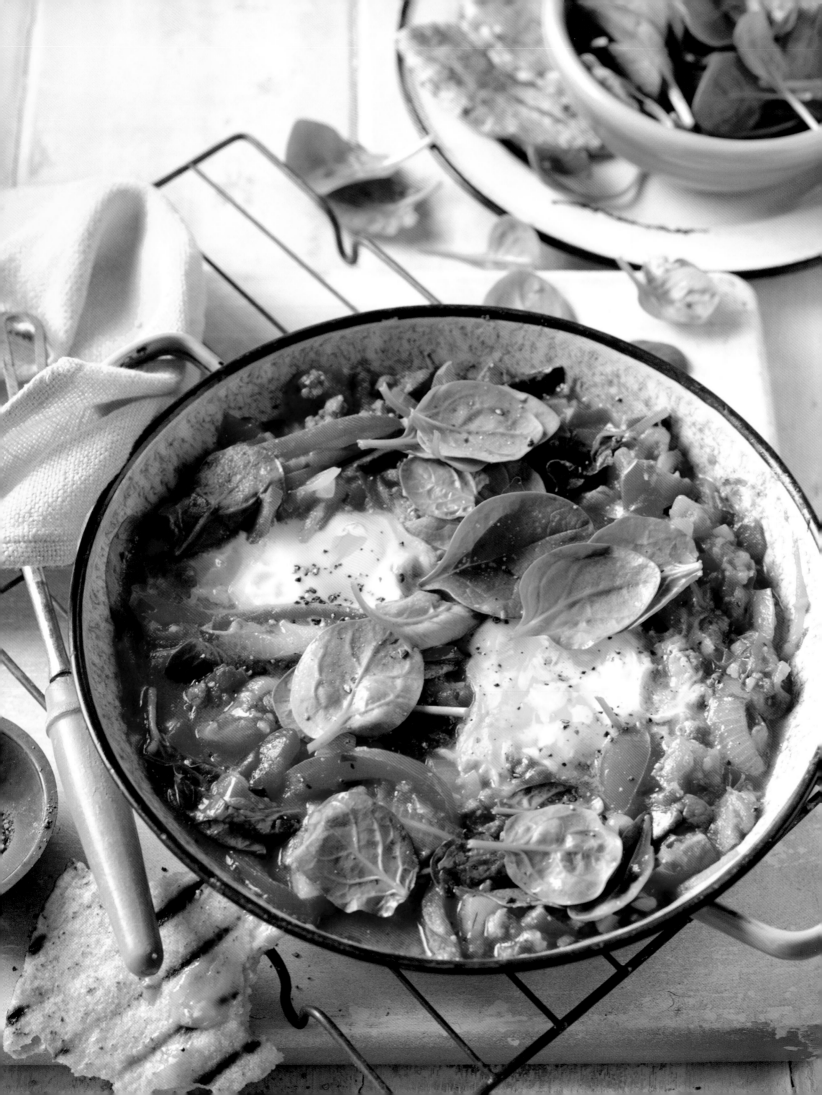

smokey shakshuka

PREP + COOK TIME 40 MINUTES ◆ **SERVES** 2

½ **teaspoon loosely packed saffron**

½ **cup (125ml) water**

½ **teaspoon cumin seeds**

3 **teaspoons rice bran oil**

1 **small brown onion (80g), sliced thinly**

2 **cloves garlic, crushed**

1 **small red capsicum (150g), sliced thinly**

100g (3 ounces) extra lean minced (ground) beef

2 **tablespoons coarsely chopped fresh flat-leaf parsley**

5 **medium vine-ripened tomatoes (750g), chopped coarsely**

½ **chipotle chilli in adobo sauce, chopped finely**

1 **teaspoon smoked paprika**

100g (3 ounces) baby spinach leaves

1 **wholemeal pitta (85g), torn crossways**

2 **small eggs**

1   Combine saffron and the water in a small jug.

2   Toast cumin seeds in a large deep dry frying pan over medium heat for 1 minute or until fragrant, remove from pan.

3   Heat 2 teaspoons of the oil in same pan; cook onion, garlic, capsicum and beef, stirring, for 5 minutes or until beef is browned and vegetables are tender.

4   Add saffron mixture, cumin, parsley, tomato, chilli and paprika to pan; bring to the boil. Reduce heat; simmer, uncovered, stirring occasionally, for 10 minutes or until mixture has thickened slightly. (If the mixture sticks to the pan while cooking, add 1 tablespoon of water to the pan to help stop the ingredients sticking.) Stir through half the spinach. Season with pepper to taste.

5   Meanwhile, heat a grill pan (or grill or barbecue) over medium heat. Rub pitta with remaining oil on both sides; cook for 1 minute each side or until charred. Remove from pan; cover to keep warm.

6   Make two indents in the hot tomato mixture with the back of a spoon. Break 1 egg into a cup, slide into indent. Repeat with remaining egg. Reduce heat to low; cook, covered, for 4 minutes or until egg whites are set.

7   Top with remaining spinach, serve with pitta.

TIPS Chipotle chilli with adobo sauce can be found in most good grocers and delicatessens. You can up the chilli for a little more heat or you can substitute chipotle chilli with 1 fresh long red chilli or ½ teaspoon dried chilli flakes if you prefer. Prepare the recipe the day before up to the end of step 4, if you like; just before serving, reheat and continue from step 5.

poached egg and avocado bruschetta

PREP + COOK TIME 20 MINUTES ◆ **SERVES** 2

1 teaspoon rice bran oil

2 teaspoons lemon juice

¼ teaspoon chilli flakes

2 tablespoons small basil leaves

2 tablespoons fresh flat-leaf parsley leaves

2 small eggs

50g (1½ ounces) baby spinach leaves

2 thick slices multigrain sourdough bread (140g)

½ clove garlic

1 medium tomato (150g), sliced thickly

½ medium avocado (125g), halved lengthways

2 teaspoons linseeds

1 To make herb salad, toss oil, juice, chilli, basil and parsley in a small bowl; season to taste with pepper.

2 Meanwhile, half fill a large shallow frying pan with water; bring to the boil. Break 1 egg into a cup, then slide into pan; repeat with remaining egg. When both eggs are in pan, return water to the boil. Cover pan, turn off heat; stand for 3 minutes or until a light film of egg white sets over yolks. Using a slotted spoon remove eggs, one at a time, from pan; drain on kitchen paper, cover to keep warm.

3 Place spinach in a heatproof bowl; cover with boiling water, drain immediately. Cool slightly then squeeze out excess liquid.

4 Toast bread, rub warm toast with garlic. Serve toast topped with spinach, tomato, avocado, egg and herb salad; sprinkle with linseeds, season with pepper. Serve immediately.

TIPS Soft boil the eggs rather than poaching them, if you like. You can use other herbs such as tarragon and chervil in this dish. Use a good quality tomato in this recipe for the best flavour.

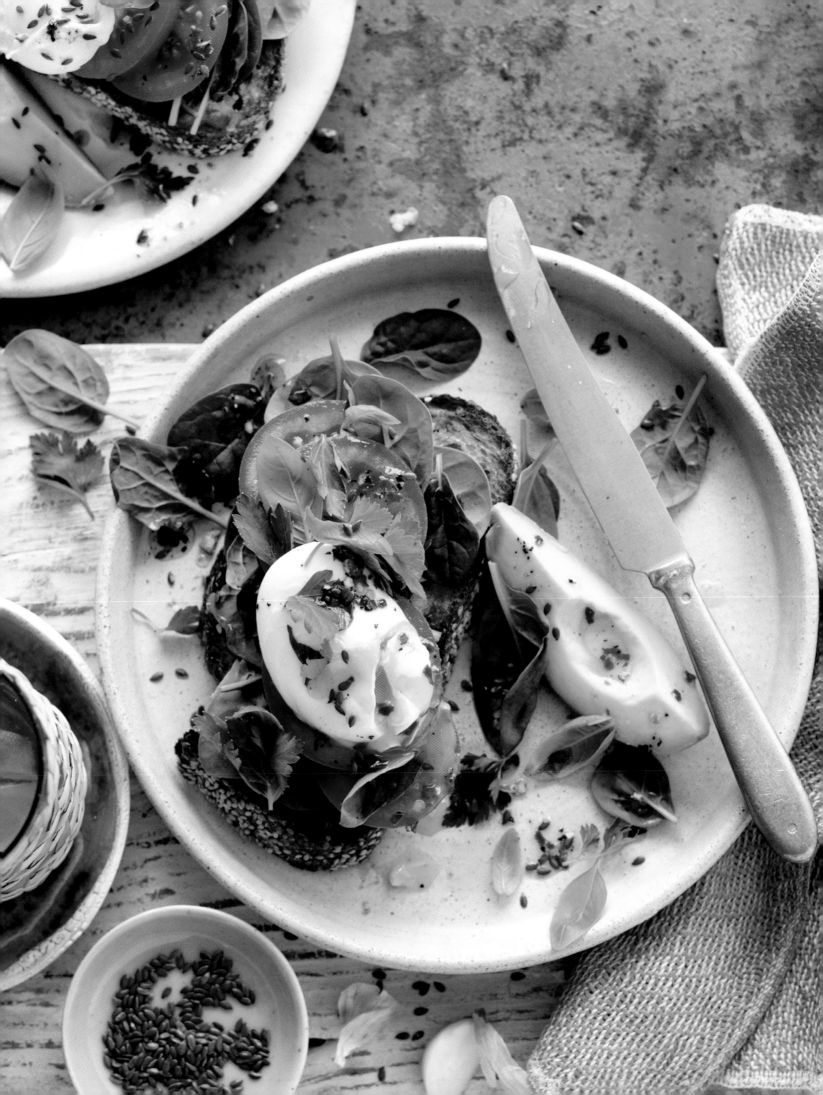

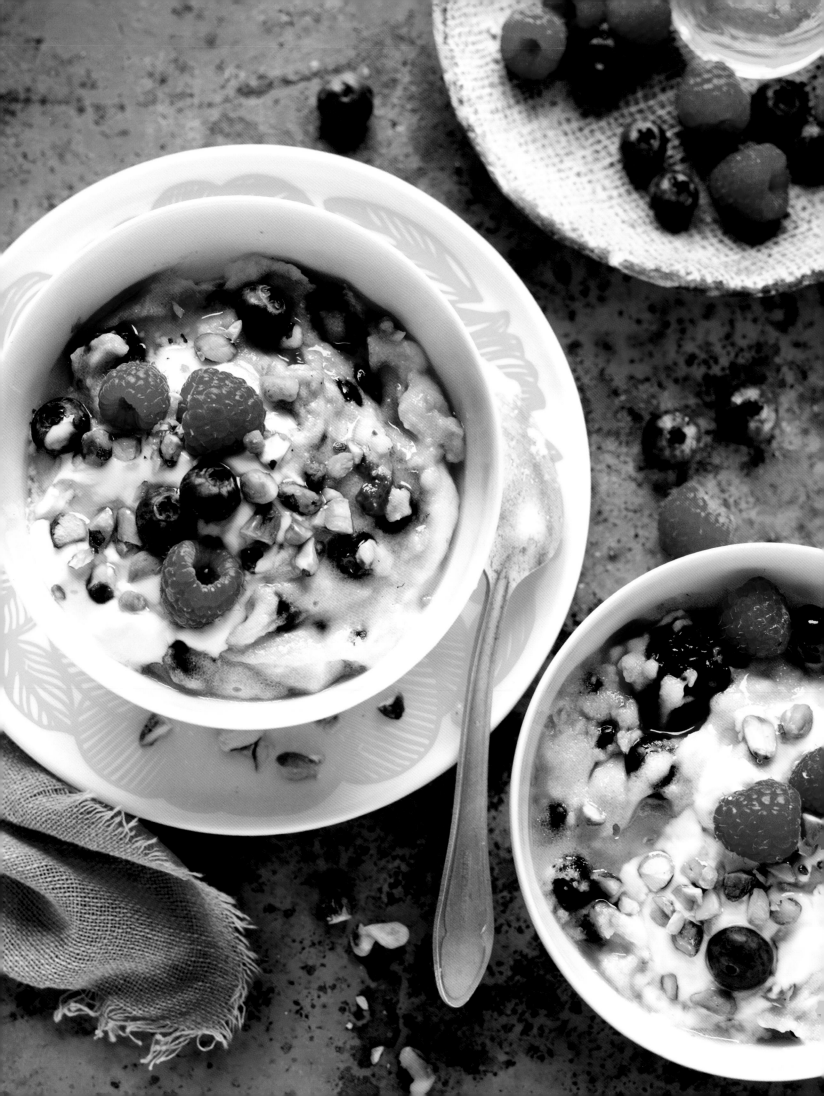

berry semolina porridge

PREP + COOK TIME 10 MINUTES ◆ SERVES 2

1 cup (250ml) skim milk

½ cup (125ml) water

1 teaspoon vanilla extract

pinch ground cinnamon

⅓ cup (55g) semolina

1 cup (150g) frozen mixed berries, thawed

¼ cup (70g) low-fat greek yoghurt

2 tablespoons chopped raw pistachios

2 teaspoons honey

1 Combine milk, the water, extract and cinnamon in a medium saucepan. Bring to the boil. Gradually add semolina. Whisk over medium heat for 2 minutes or until thick. Remove from heat; stir in ⅔ cup berries.

2 Divide porridge into serving bowls. Top with yoghurt, nuts, honey and remaining berries.

TIP Use your favourite nuts in this recipe to add crunch and fibre.

NUTRITIONAL COUNT PER SERVING

- 24g total fat
- 6.8g saturated fat
- 1758kJ (420 cal)
- 30.3g carbohydrate
- 15.9g protein
- 7.7g fibre
- 402mg sodium
- low GI

pea fritters with avocado goat's cheese

PREP + COOK TIME 20 MINUTES ◆ SERVES 2

½ cup (75g) wholemeal self-raising flour

1 teaspoon finely grated lemon rind

1 small egg

½ cup (125ml) skim milk

1 cup (120g) frozen peas, thawed

1 teaspoon rice bran oil

1 small avocado (200g)

30g (1 ounces) fresh goat's cheese, crumbled

2 tablespoons chopped fresh mint leaves

30g (1 ounce) rocket leaves (arugula)

80g (2½ ounces) chopped cherry tomatoes, quartered

2 lemon wedges

1 Combine sifted flour and rind in a medium bowl. Add egg and milk, whisk to combine. Fold through peas. Season with pepper.

2 Heat oil in a large, non-stick frying pan over medium heat; cook ⅓-cups of batter, in batches, for 3 minutes each side or until browned lightly and cooked through. Cover to keep warm.

3 Meanwhile, mash avocado in a small bowl with a fork. Stir through cheese and mint. Serve fritters with avocado mash, rocket, tomato and wedges.

TIPS Thaw peas by running under boiling water. The mixture is quite loose, it will spread once in the pan.

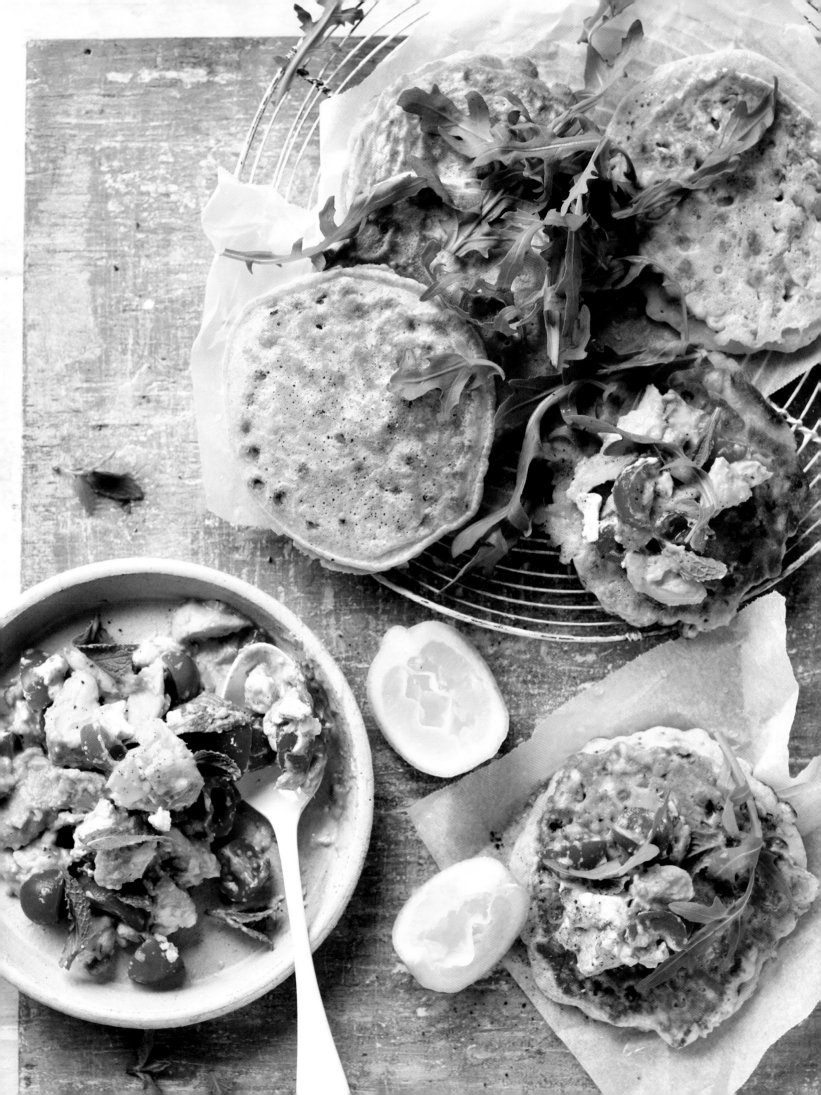

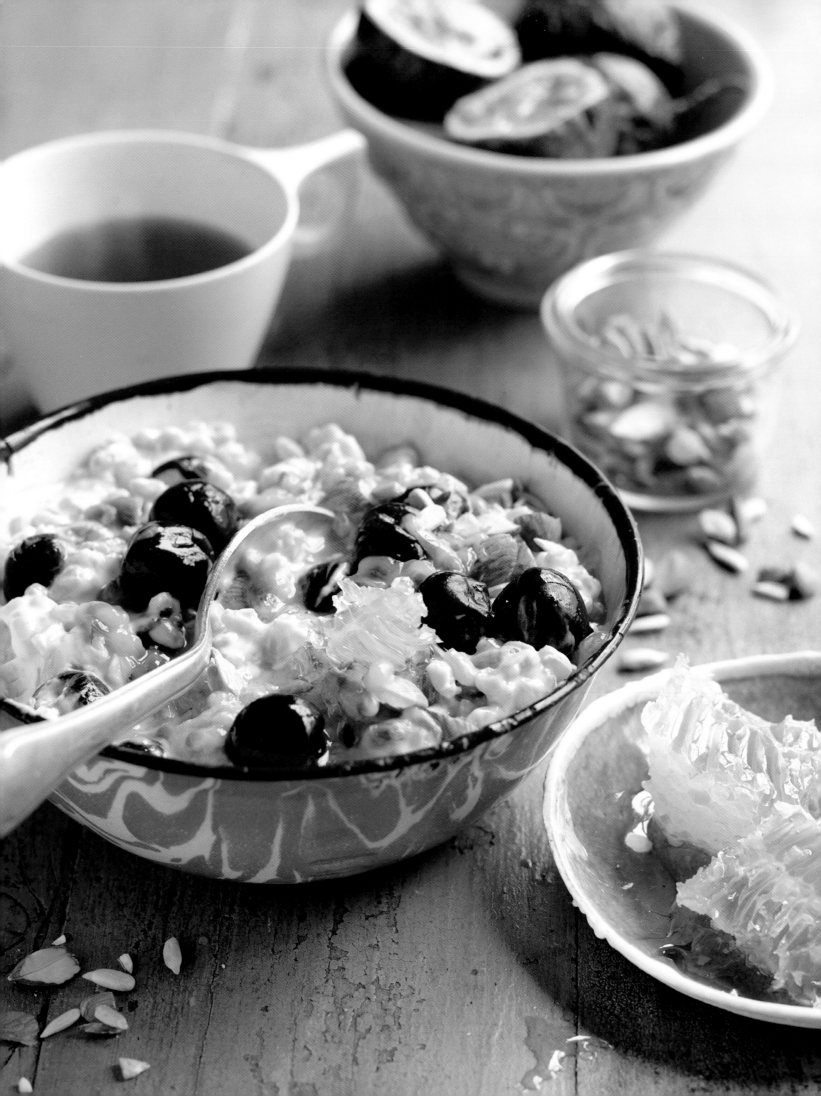

NUTRITIONAL COUNT PER SERVING

● 16.8g total fat   ● 17.3g protein

● 4.7g saturated fat   ● 12g fibre

● 2092kJ (500 cal)   ● 116mg sodium

● 62.5g carbohydrate   ● low GI

pearl barley and cherry breakfast bowl

PREP + COOK TIME 50 MINUTES ◆ SERVES 2

½ cup (100g) pearl barley

1½ cups (375ml) water

1 cup (280g) sheep's milk yoghurt

1½ cups (185g) frozen pitted cherries, thawed

2 tablespoons fresh passionfruit pulp

30g (1 ounce) fresh honeycomb, sliced

1 tablespoon chopped fresh mint leaves

2 tablespoons coarsely chopped natural almonds

1 tablespoon sunflower seeds

1   Combine barley and the water in a small saucepan over high heat, bring to the boil; reduce heat to low, cover, simmer for 35 minutes or until tender. Drain; rinse under cold water until cool.

2   Combine barley, yoghurt and ⅔ cup of the cherries in a medium bowl. Divide into serving bowls. Top with remaining cherries, passionfruit, honeycomb, mint, nuts and sunflower seeds.

TIPS You could also try this with cooked quinoa instead of barley. This recipe can be prepared the day before up to the end of step 1. Frozen raspberries can be used instead of cherries.

NUTRITIONAL COUNT PER SERVING

- 21.8g total fat
- 5.9g saturated fat
- 2227kJ (532 cal)
- 61.4g carbohydrate
- 17.1g protein
- 10.3g fibre
- 80mg sodium
- low GI

baked pina colada granola

PREP + COOK TIME 40 MINUTES ◆ SERVES 2

1 herbal lemon tea bag

¼ cup (60ml) boiling water

1½ cups (135g) rolled oats

2 tablespoons chopped pecans

2 tablespoons sunflower seeds

¼ cup (10g) coconut flakes

¼ cup (40g) chopped dried pineapple

1 cup (250ml) skim milk

1 Preheat oven to 160°C/325°F. Line a large oven tray with baking paper.

2 Combine tea bag and the boiling water in a small heatproof bowl. Stand for 5 minutes. Discard tea bag.

3 Combine oats, nuts and sunflower seeds on tray. Drizzle with tea, stir to coat. Bake for 10 minutes. Stir and bake for a further 10 minutes. Add coconut; bake for 3 minutes or until golden.

4 Stir through pineapple. Cool muesli on tray. Divide into serving bowls. Pour over milk.

TIP Recipe can be doubled and stored in an airtight container; it will last for months if stored correctly.

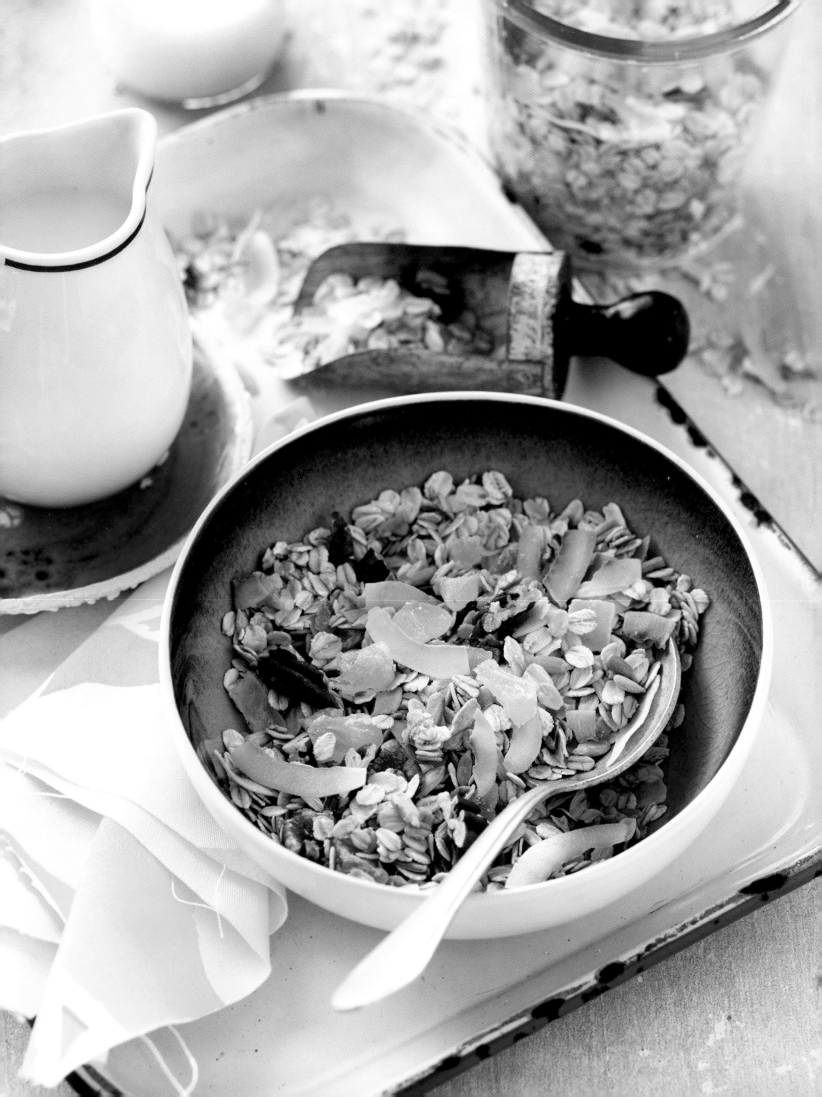

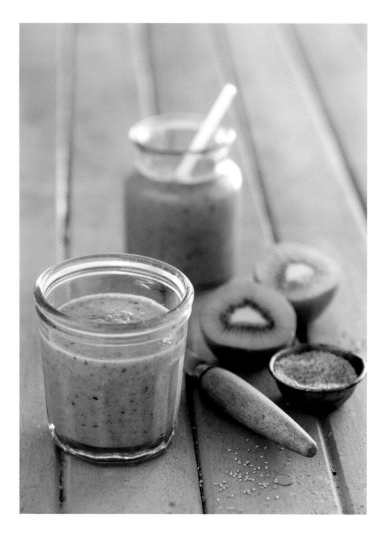

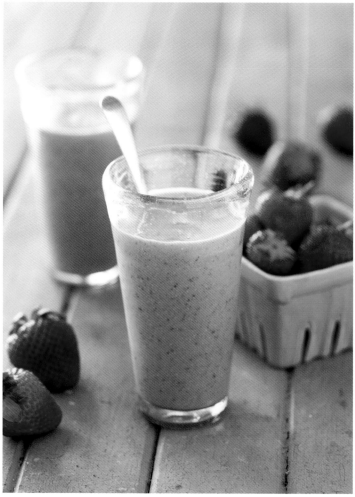

green smoothie

PREP + COOK TIME 10 MINUTES ◆ **SERVES** 2

Roughly chop 1 medium banana and 2 kiwi fruit. Blend or process fruit with 30g (1 ounce) baby spinach leaves, 1 cup almond milk, 1 tablespoon honey and 2 teaspoons chia seeds until smooth.

TIP Chia seeds are available from supermarkets and health food stores. They come in black or white varieties and either type would work in this recipe. You could omit the chia seeds if you like.

pb & j smoothie

PREP + COOK TIME 5 MINUTES ◆ **SERVES** 2

Blend 1½ cups frozen strawberries, 1½ tablespoons smooth light peanut butter, 2 tablespoons wheat germ, 1 tablespoon brown rice malt syrup and 1½ cups low-fat milk until smooth.

TIP You could also use honey or agave syrup instead of the brown rice malt syrup.

NUTRITIONAL COUNT PER SERVING

- 15.6g total fat
- 1g saturated fat
- 1297kJ (310 cal)
- 32.6g carbohydrate
- 7.3g protein
- 7.1g fibre
- 12mg sodium
- low GI

NUTRITIONAL COUNT PER SERVING

- 10.3g total fat
- 1.8g saturated fat
- 1260kJ (301 cal)
- 33.7g carbohydrate
- 15.8g protein
- 5.9g fibre
- 234mg sodium
- low GI

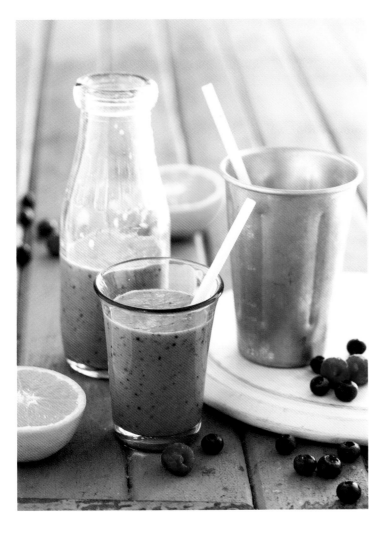

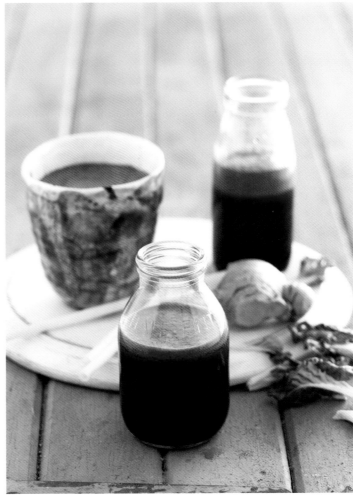

orange berry smoothie

PREP + COOK TIME 10 MINUTES ◆ MAKES 2

Roughly chop 1 medium peeled orange and 1 medium cored pear. Blend or process fruit with 1 cup frozen mixed berries, 150g (4½ ounces) low-fat, low-sugar vanilla yoghurt and ¼ cup pomegranate juice until smooth.

TIP Use apple juice instead of the pomegranate juice, if you prefer.

invigorating fruit & vegetable juice

PREP + COOK TIME 10 MINUTES SERVES 2

Push 2 coarsely chopped large beetroot, 2 trimmed celery stalks, 130g (4 ounces) silver beet leaves (swiss chard), 2 chopped large green apples, 1 cup fresh flat-leaf parsley, 1 segmented medium lemon and 20g (¾-ounce) peeled fresh ginger through a juice extractor into a jug. Stir; serve immediately.

TIP Have the fruit washed and chopped, and on hand in the refrigerator to save time; juice just before serving to retain the nutrients in the fruit and vegetables.

NUTRITIONAL COUNT PER SERVING

- 0.4g total fat
- 0.1g saturated fat
- 862kJ (206 cal)
- 38.9g carbohydrate
- 6.4g protein
- 9.4g fibre
- 62mg sodium
- low GI

NUTRITIONAL COUNT PER SERVING

- 0.8g total fat
- 0g saturated fat
- 917kJ (219 cal)
- 37.8g carbohydrate
- 7.3g protein
- 2.4g fibre
- 370mg sodium
- low GI

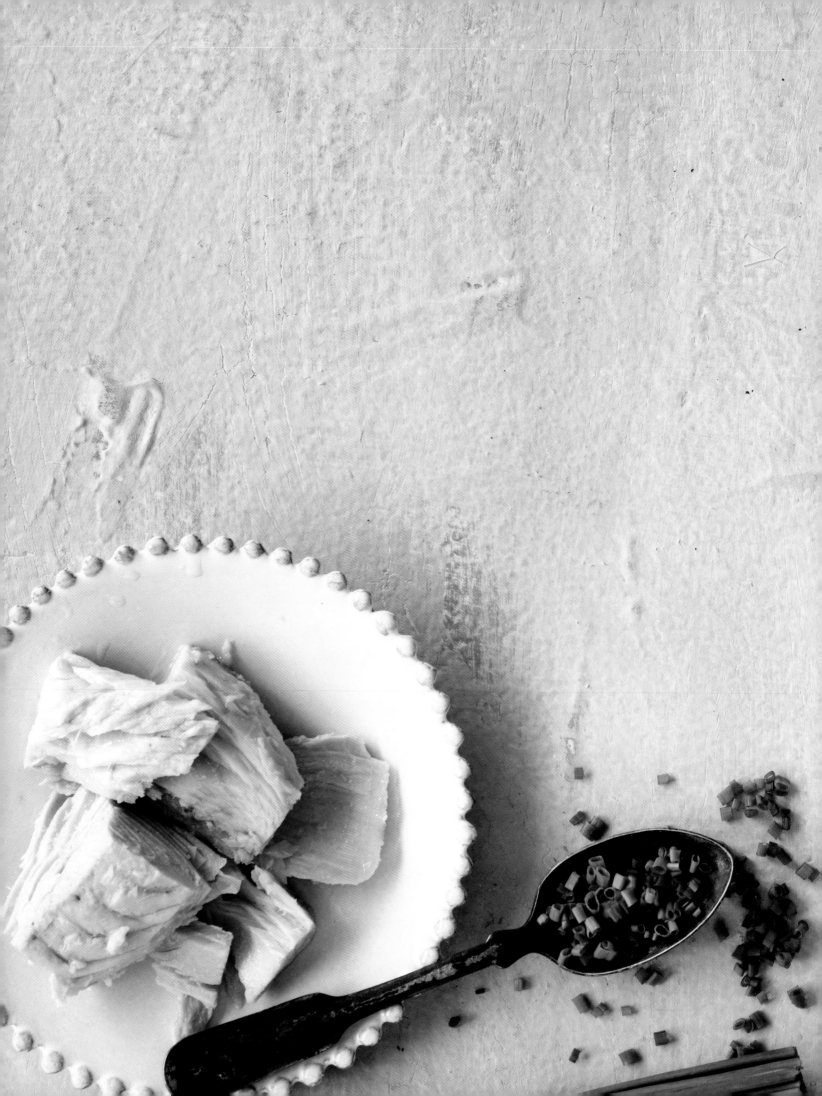

LUNCH

Skipping lunch, but having a snack, is not good for blood sugar control; eat regular meals throughout the day.

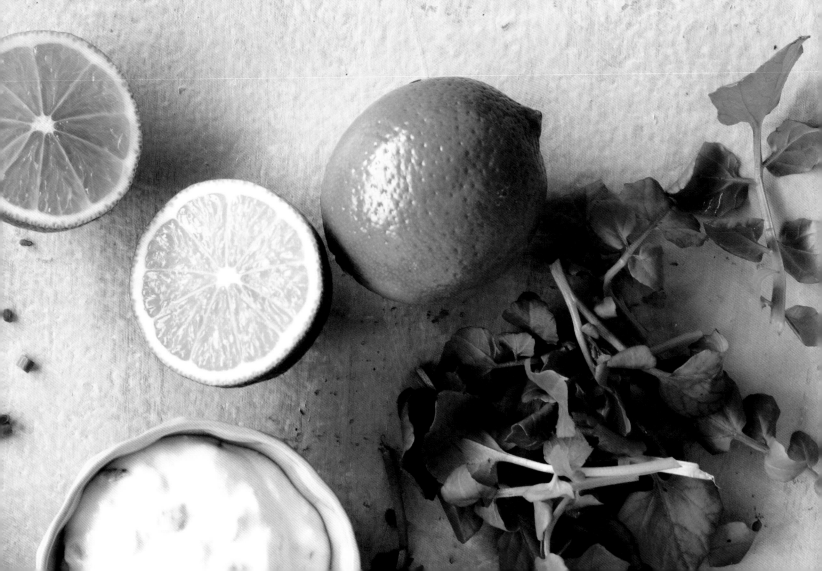

asian-style chicken salad

PREP + COOK TIME 15 MINUTES ◆ SERVES 2

100g (3 ounces) soba noodles

1½ cups (240g) shredded cooked skinless chicken breast

6 iceberg lettuce leaves, torn

1 lebanese cucumber (130g), sliced thinly

½ small red onion (50g), sliced thinly

1 large mandarin (250g), segmented

1 small avocado (200g), chopped coarsely

2 teaspoons sesame seeds, toasted

ASIAN DRESSING

2 tablespoons rice wine vinegar

1 tablespoon fresh mandarin juice

2 teaspoons salt-reduced soy sauce

1 teaspoon grated fresh ginger

½ teaspoon sesame oil

1 Make asian dressing.

2 Cook noodles in a large saucepan of boiling water until tender; drain. Rinse under cold water; drain.

3 Combine all ingredients in a large bowl. Drizzle with dressing.

ASIAN DRESSING Combine ingredients in a small bowl.

TIPS You can use store-bought barbecue chicken, leftover roast chicken, or just bake or poach two small chicken breasts. Swap the soba noodles for rice or egg noodles.

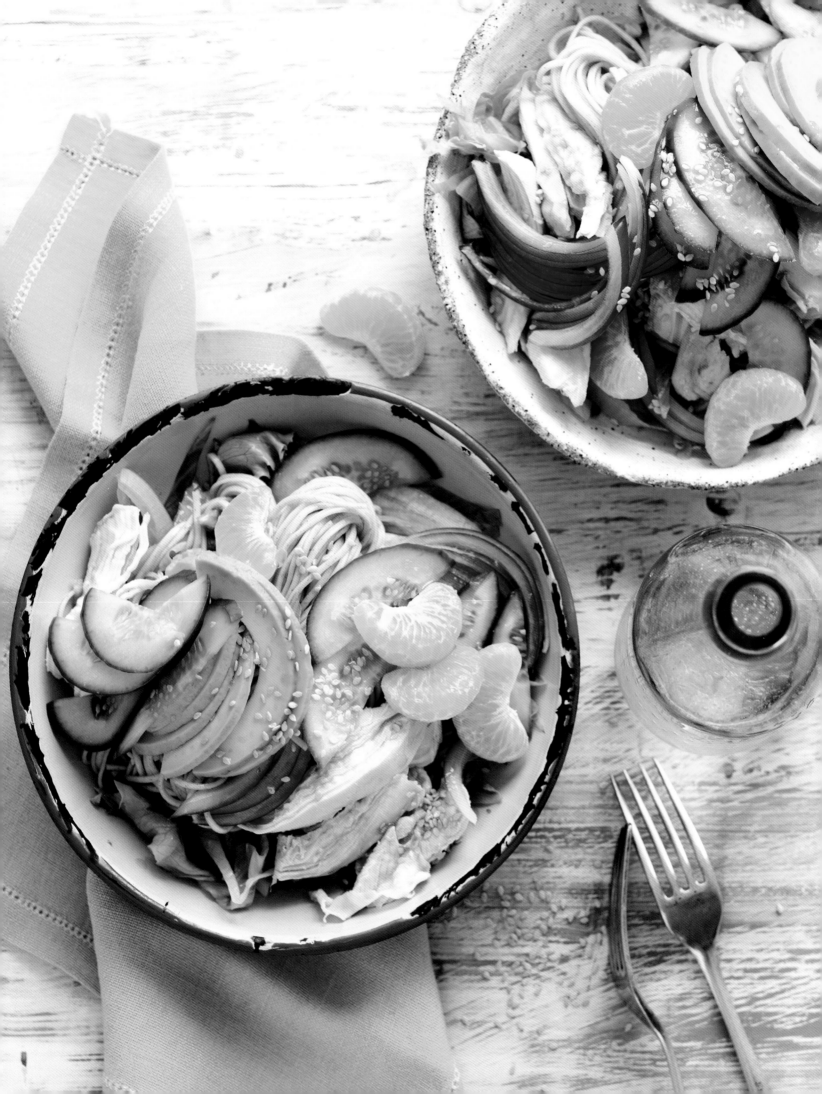

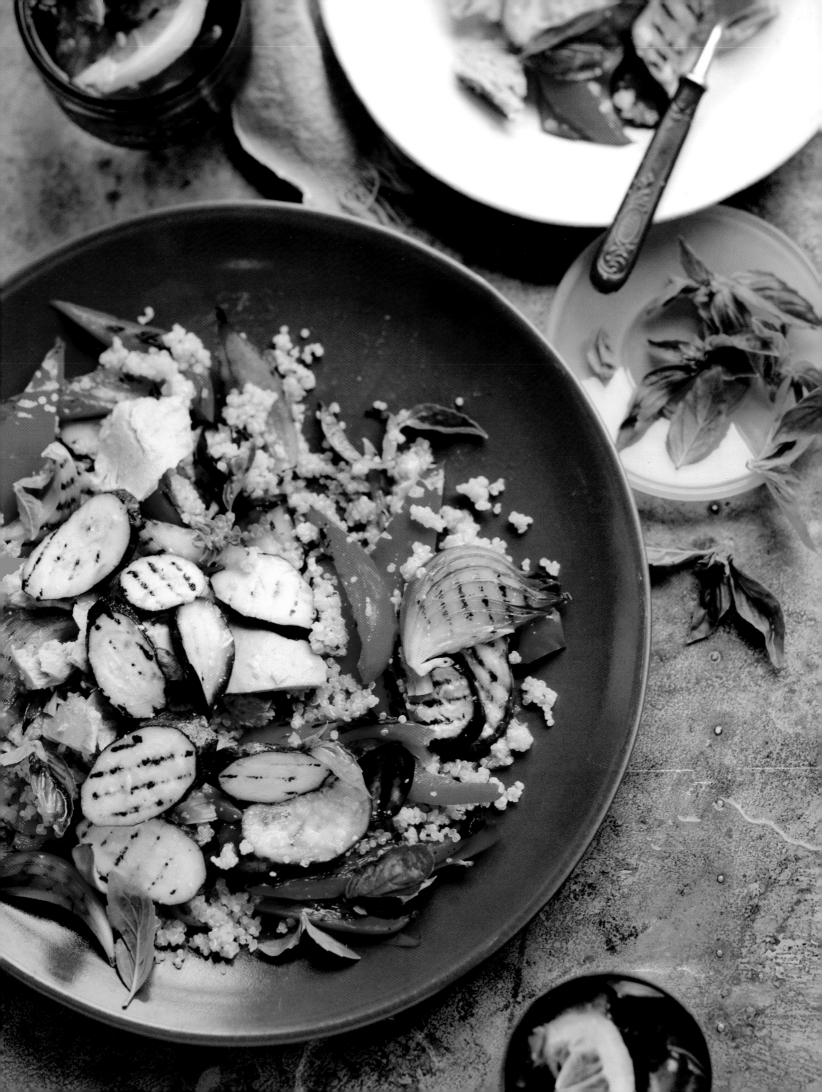

NUTRITIONAL COUNT PER SERVING

● 9.1g total fat   ● 26g protein
● 1.7g saturated fat ● 5.8g fibre
● 1332kJ (318 cal)   ● 118g sodium
● 28.9g carbohydrate ● low GI

quinoa salad with char-grilled vegetables and tuna

PREP + COOK TIME 25 MINUTES ◆ SERVES 2

1 small red capsicum (bell pepper) (150g), quartered

1 medium zucchini (120g), sliced thinly

1 baby eggplant (60g), sliced thinly

1 small red onion (100g), cut into wedges

⅓ cup (70g) quinoa, rinsed, drained

⅔ cup (160ml) water

2 teaspoons olive oil

¼ cup (60ml) lemon juice

1 teaspoon dijon mustard

185g (6½ ounces) canned tuna in springwater, drained

2 tablespoons baby basil leaves

1 Cook capsicum, zucchini, eggplant and onion on a heated oiled grill plate (or grill or barbecue) until tender. Slice capsicum thickly.

2 Meanwhile, place quinoa in a small saucepan with the water; bring to the boil. Reduce heat to low; simmer, covered, for 15 minutes or until tender and water is absorbed. Remove from heat; stand for 10 minutes, then fluff with a fork.

3 Combine oil, juice and mustard in a screw-top jar; shake well.

4 Place quinoa, vegetables and tuna in a bowl with dressing; toss gently to combine. Serve topped with basil leaves.

TIPS Vegetables can be grilled a day ahead; store, covered, in the fridge. The salad can be served warm or cold; add some rocket (arugula) or spinach leaves, if you like.

NUTRITIONAL COUNT PER SERVING

● 2.7g total fat   ● 12g protein
● 0.5g saturated fat   ● 6.7g fibre
● 877kJ (209 cal)   ● 296mg sodium
● 30.9g carbohydrate   ● low GI

spiced lentil and roasted kumara soup

PREP + COOK TIME 45 MINUTES ◆ **SERVES** 2

1 small kumara (orange sweet potato) (250g), cut into 2cm (¾-inch) cubes

cooking-oil spray

1 small brown onion (80g), chopped coarsely

1 clove garlic, crushed

½ cup (125ml) salt-reduced vegetable stock

½ teaspoon each ground cumin and coriander

¼ teaspoon turmeric

¼ cup (50g) dried red lentils, rinsed, drained

2 cups (500ml) water

⅓ cup (95g) low-fat plain yoghurt

2 tablespoons finely chopped fresh coriander (cilantro)

1 Preheat oven to 220°C/425°F. Place kumara on a baking-paper-lined oven tray; spray with oil. Bake for 25 minutes until golden and tender.

2 Meanwhile, cook onion, garlic and 2 tablespoons of the stock in a medium saucepan over high heat, stirring, for 3 minutes or until onion is tender. Add spices; cook, stirring, for 30 seconds or until fragrant. Stir in lentils, remaining stock and the water; bring to the boil. Reduce heat; simmer, uncovered, for 15 minutes or until lentils are tender. Add kumara. Cook for 5 minutes. Cool mixture 10 minutes.

3 Blend or process mixture until smooth. Return mixture to pan; stir until hot.

4 Combine yoghurt and coriander in a small bowl. Serve soup topped with yoghurt mixture and extra coriander leaves, if you like.

TIPS Soup can be made a day ahead; store, covered, in the fridge. Freeze the soup without the yoghurt mixture in an airtight container for up to 3 months. Defrost in the fridge overnight and reheat in a small saucepan on the stove over medium heat for about 10 minutes or until hot.

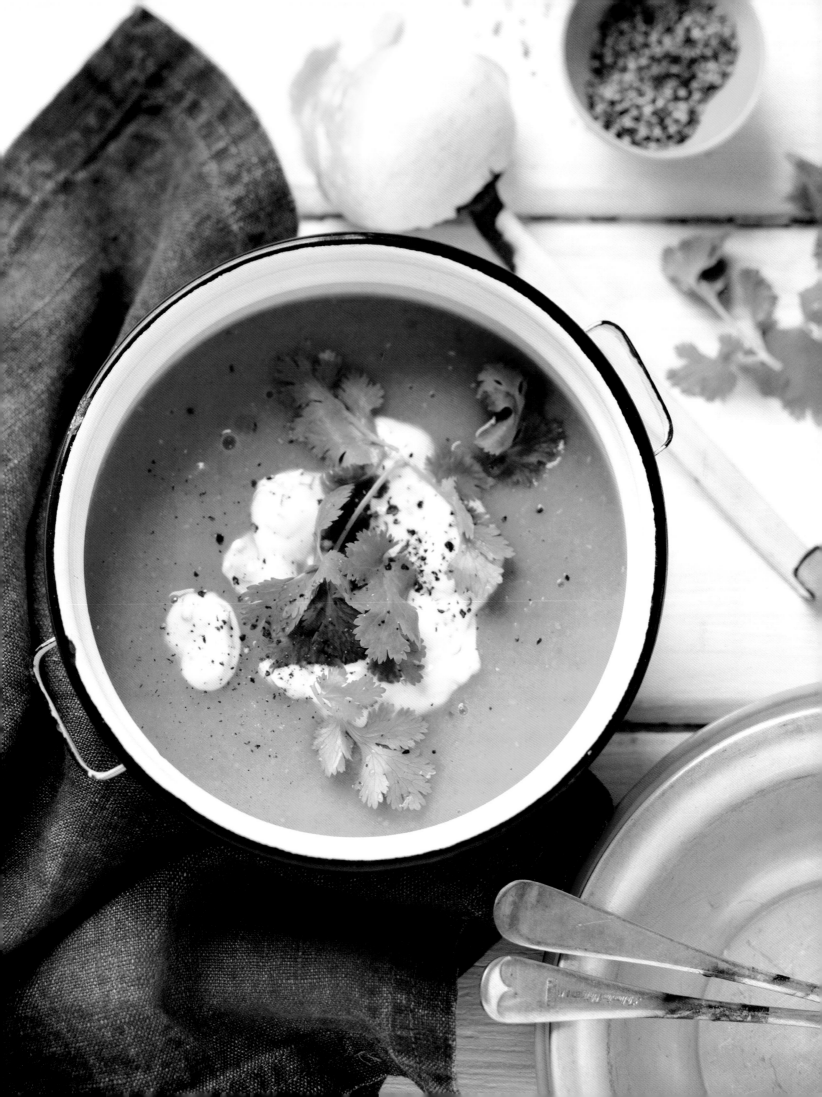

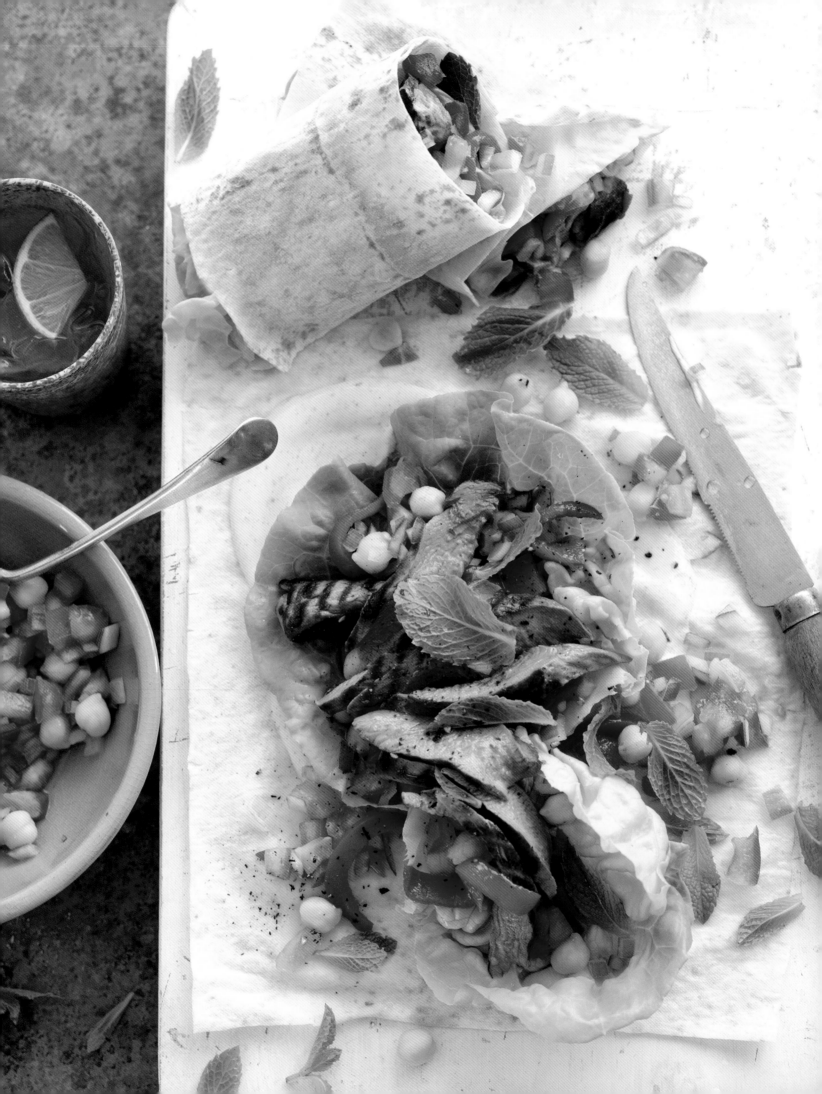

NUTRITIONAL COUNT PER SERVING

- 9.9g total fat
- 2.6g saturated fat
- 1593kJ (381 cal)
- 34.8g carbohydrate
- 33.3g protein
- 5.9g fibre
- 389mg sodium
- low GI

moroccan lamb and chickpea wraps

PREP + COOK TIME 15 MINUTES ◆ **SERVES** 2

200g (6 ounces) lamb fillets

125g (4 ounces) canned chickpeas (garbanzo beans), rinsed, drained

60g (2 ounces) drained char-grilled capsicum (bell pepper), sliced thinly

½ small red onion (50g), chopped finely

1 large tomato, chopped finely

¼ cup loosely packed fresh mint leaves

2 tablespoons lemon juice

1 teaspoon olive oil

¼ cup (70g) low-fat plain yoghurt

¼ teaspoon harissa paste

6 butter (boston) lettuce leaves

2 rye mountain breads (50g)

1 Cook lamb on a heated oiled grill plate (or grill or barbecue) until cooked as desired. Cover lamb; rest for 5 minutes, then slice thickly.

2 Meanwhile, combine chickpeas, capsicum, onion, tomato, mint, juice and oil in a bowl; stir to combine.

3 Combine yoghurt and harissa in a small bowl.

4 Divide yoghurt mixture, lettuce, lamb and chickpea mixture between wraps. Roll firmly to enclose filling.

TIPS There are many types of mountain bread available; choose your favourite for this recipe. Harissa is a very hot paste; there are many different brands of harissa paste available, and the strengths vary enormously. Reduce the amount of harissa to suit your taste if you are not used to the fiery heat.

asian beef rolls

PREP TIME 15 MINUTES ◆ **SERVES** 2

1 tablespoon smooth salt-reduced peanut butter

1 teaspoon salt-reduced soy sauce

1 tablespoon boiling water

2 long wholegrain bread rolls (100g), split

60g (2 ounces) thinly sliced salt-reduced rare roast beef

4 butter (boston) lettuce leaves

1 small carrot (70g), sliced thinly

4 long sprigs fresh coriander leaves (cilantro)

1 green onion (scallion), halved crossways

½ fresh long red chilli, sliced thinly

1 Combine peanut butter, sauce and the water in a small bowl. Spread over the inside of bread rolls.

2 Sandwich beef, lettuce, carrot, coriander, green onion and chilli between rolls. Serve with a squeeze of lime, if you like.

TIP You could use left-over roast beef or char-grill a beef rump steak.

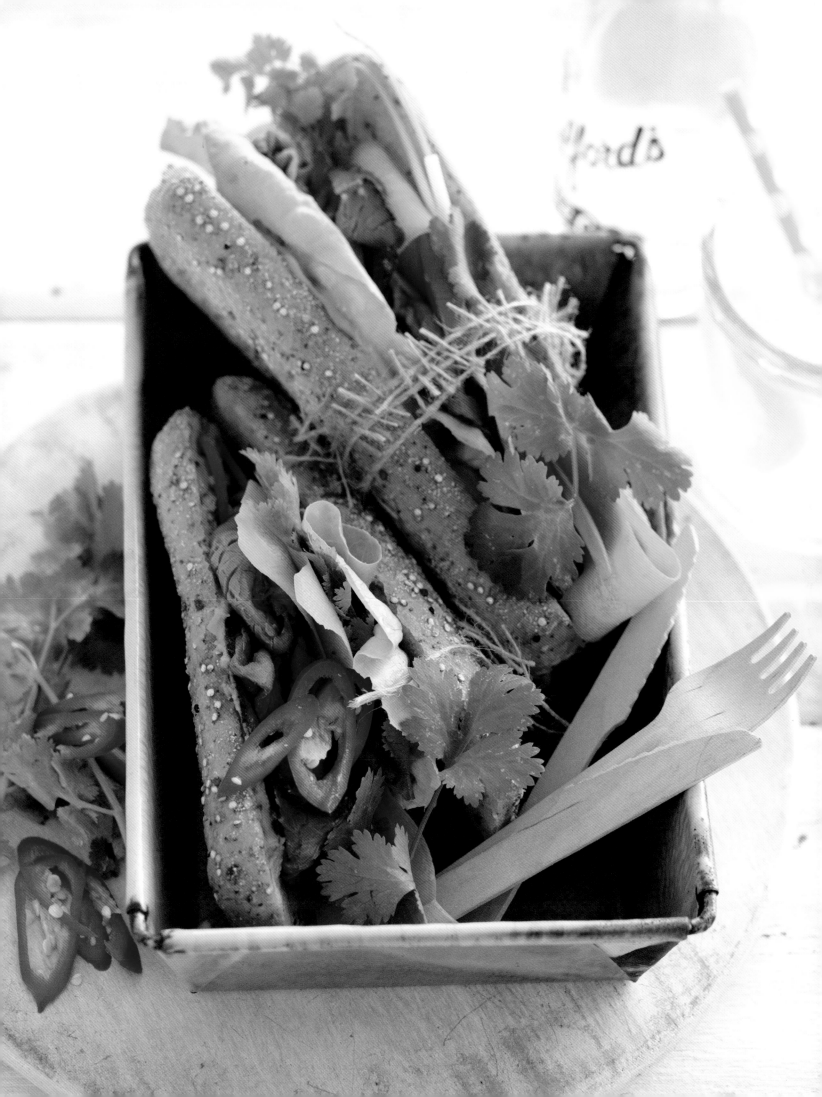

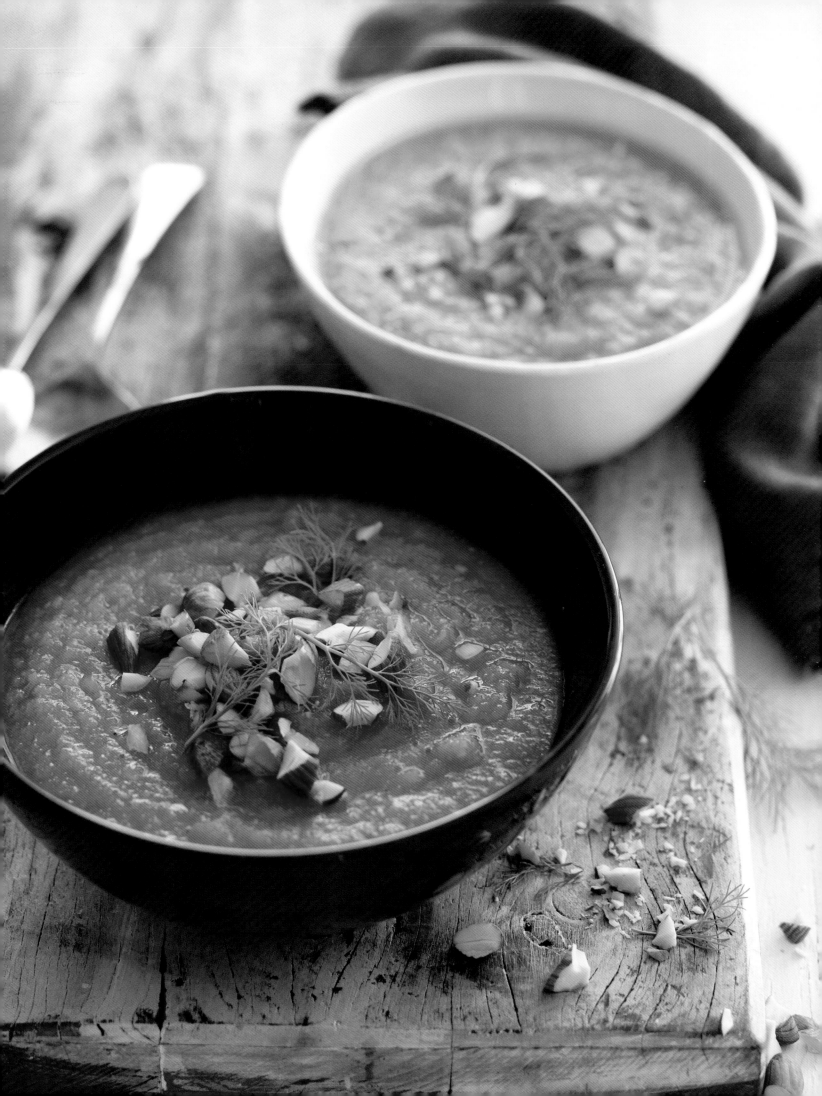

tomato and fennel soup

PREP + COOK TIME 50 MINUTES ◆ SERVES 2

1 large fennel bulb (550g)

1 small kumara (orange sweet potato) (250g), cut into 2cm (¾-inch) pieces

4 small tomatoes (360g), halved

1 medium red onion (170g), cut into wedges

2 cloves garlic, unpeeled

cooking-oil spray

2½ cups (625ml) salt-reduced vegetable stock

⅓ cup (55g) natural almonds, chopped coarsely

1 Preheat oven to 200°C/400°F. Line a large oven tray with baking paper.

2 Trim fennel, reserving 1 tablespoon of fennel fronds; cut fennel into wedges. Combine fennel, kumara, tomato, onion and garlic on tray. Lightly spray with oil. Roast 30 minutes or until tender and browned.

3 Peel garlic; blend or process kumara, tomato, fennel, onion, garlic and stock until smooth.

4 Place the soup in a medium saucepan. Bring to the boil. Serve soup sprinkled with nuts and reserved fennel fronds.

TIP Make the soup ahead of time and freeze for up to 3 months or refrigerate for 1 week.

turkey and brown rice salad

PREP + COOK TIME 40 MINUTES ◆ SERVES 2

⅔ cup (130g) brown rice

100g (3 ounces) green beans, trimmed, halved lengthways

200g (6½ ounces) turkey breast steaks

3 red radishes (105g), sliced thinly

1 lebanese cucumber (130g), halved, sliced thinly

40g (1½ ounces) goat's cheese, crumbled

2 green onions (scallions), sliced thinly

1 trimmed celery stalk (100g), sliced thinly

1 tablespoon cashews, toasted, coarsely chopped

50g (1½ ounces) baby rocket leaves (arugula)

¼ cup loosely packed torn fresh basil leaves

1 tablespoon olive oil

2 tablespoons lemon juice

1   Place rice in a medium saucepan, cover with water; bring to the boil. Reduce heat; simmer, uncovered, for 35 minutes or until tender. Drain; rinse under cold water. Drain well.

2   Meanwhile, cook beans in a small saucepan of boiling water for 3 minutes or until just tender. Drain; refresh under cold water, drain.

3   Cook turkey on a heated oiled grill pan (or grill or barbecue) for 3 minutes each side or until cooked through. Cover; rest for 5 minutes, then slice thickly.

4   Combine rice with beans, turkey, radish, cucumber, cheese, onion, celery, nuts, rocket and basil in a large bowl. Drizzle with combined oil and juice; toss to combine.

TIPS This recipe is perfect for any lunchbox as you can make it the night before; store, covered, in the fridge. If you're short of time, try making this salad with quinoa instead of rice; it will take less than half the time to cook and has a great fibre content, just like brown rice. You could use chicken breast or lamb fillets instead of the turkey.

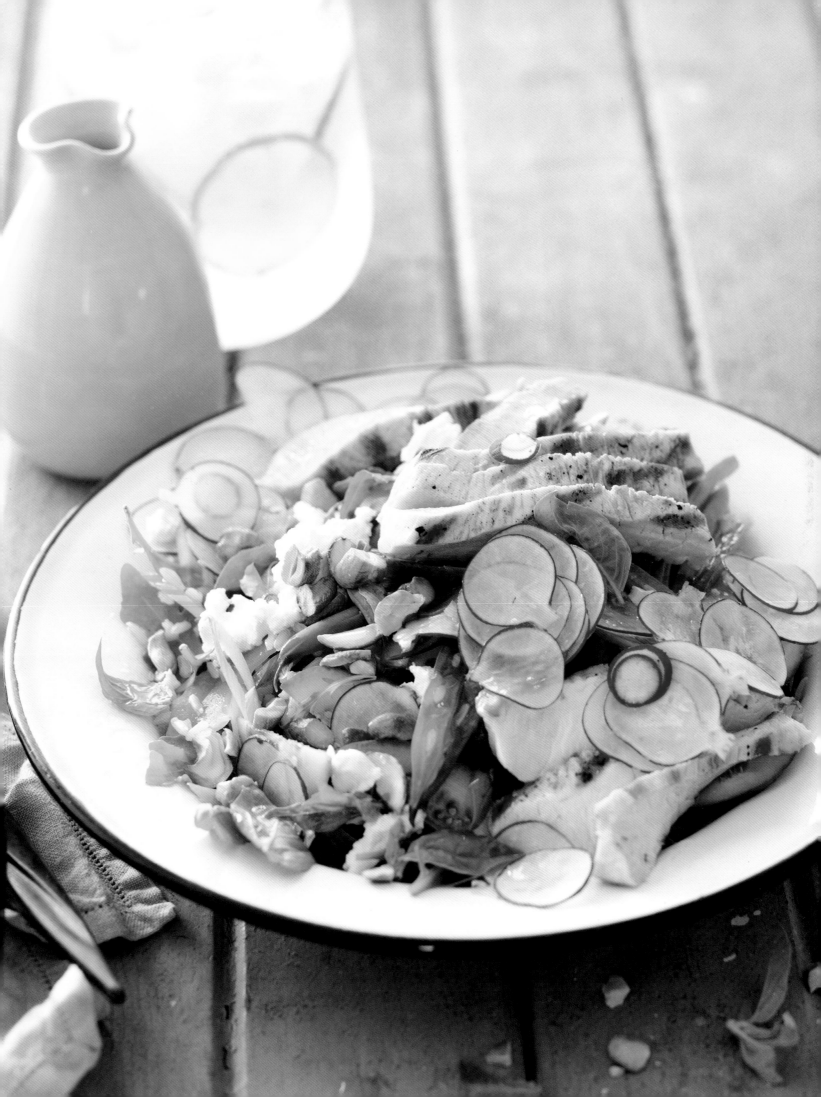

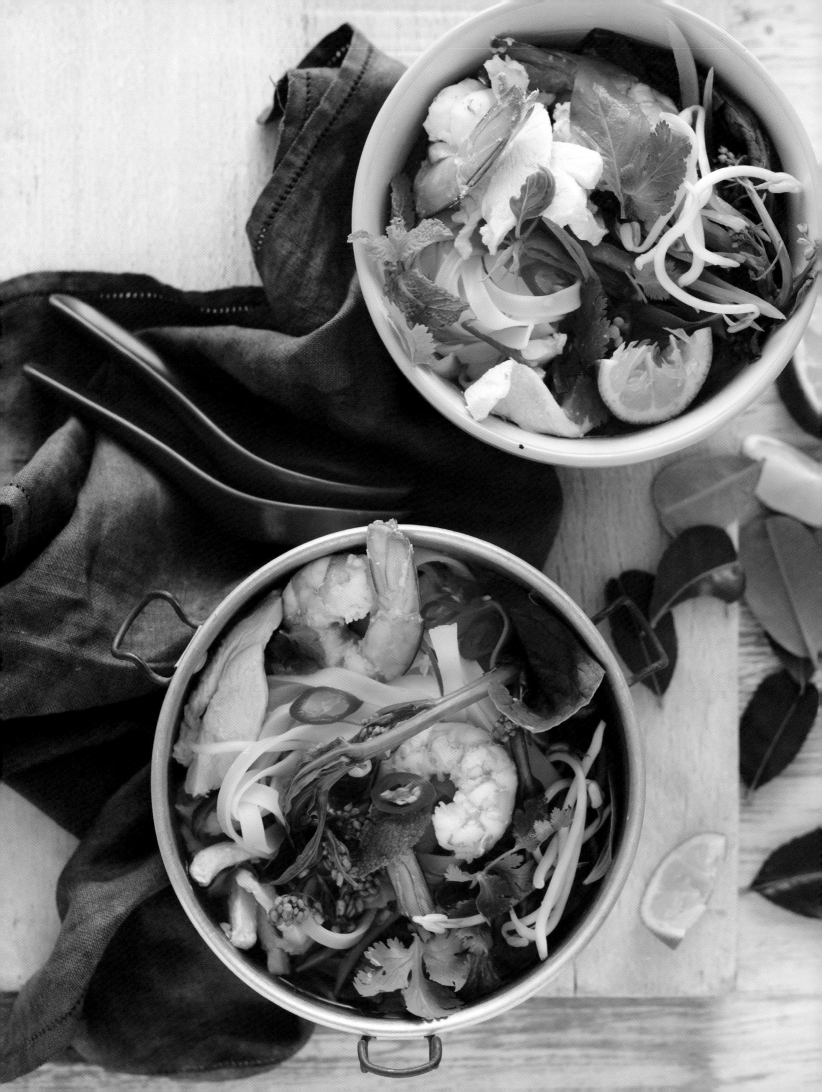

hot and sour prawn and chicken soup

PREP + COOK TIME 30 MINUTES ◆ SERVES 2

3 cups (750ml) water

4 fresh kaffir lime leaves, torn

40g (¾ ounce) fresh ginger, sliced thickly

1 fresh small red thai (serrano) chilli, sliced thinly

100g (3 ounces) dried rice noodles

4 green king prawns (shrimp) (140g)

100g (3 ounces) chicken breast, sliced thinly

1 tablespoon lime juice

100g (3 ounces) snow peas, shredded

350g (8 ounces) baby choy sum, trimmed, chopped coarsely

½ cup (40g) bean sprouts

¼ cup each loosely packed fresh coriander (cilantro), mint and thai basil leaves

1 Combine the water, lime leaves, ginger and half the chilli in a medium saucepan over high heat; bring to the boil. Reduce heat; simmer, covered, for 10 minutes; discard leaves and ginger.

2 Meanwhile, cook noodles in a medium saucepan of boiling water according to packet directions; drain.

3 Shell and devein prawns leaving tails intact. Add prawns and chicken to broth; simmer for 3 minutes or until chicken and prawns are cooked. Stir in lime juice.

4 Divide noodles, snow peas and choy sum between two serving bowls; ladle broth mixture over top. Top with sprouts, herbs and remaining chilli.

TIPS Make sure the broth is piping hot so it will slightly cook the choy sum and snow peas. If you can't find baby choy sum, use half a bunch of normal choy sum or another asian green. Kaffir lime leaves are sold in small packets. Freeze the remaining leaves – they lose a bit of colour but keep their flavour. You can use a packaged salt-reduced chicken stock instead of the water, if you like.

vegetable rösti with smoked salmon and sour cream

PREP + COOK TIME 30 MINUTES ◆ SERVES 2

½ small kumara (orange sweet potato) (125g), peeled, grated coarsely

2 shallots (50g), sliced finely

1 medium silver beet leaf (swiss chard) (65g), trimmed, shredded

1 small zucchini (90g), grated coarsely

1 egg, beaten lightly

⅓ cup (50g) wholemeal spelt flour

1 tablespoon olive oil

120g (4 ounces) smoked salmon

1½ tablespoons light sour cream

1 tablespoon fresh dill sprigs

1 Combine kumara, shallot, silver beet, zucchini, egg and flour in a large bowl; mix well. Divide mixture into four equal portions.

2 Heat oil in a large non-stick frying pan over medium heat, place kumara mixture into pan; press each portion down with a spatula to flatten. Cook 4 minutes each side or until rösti are golden and cooked through.

3 Serve rösti topped with smoked salmon, sour cream and dill.

TIP Cooked rosti can be stored in the refrigerator overnight and reheated in a sandwich press.

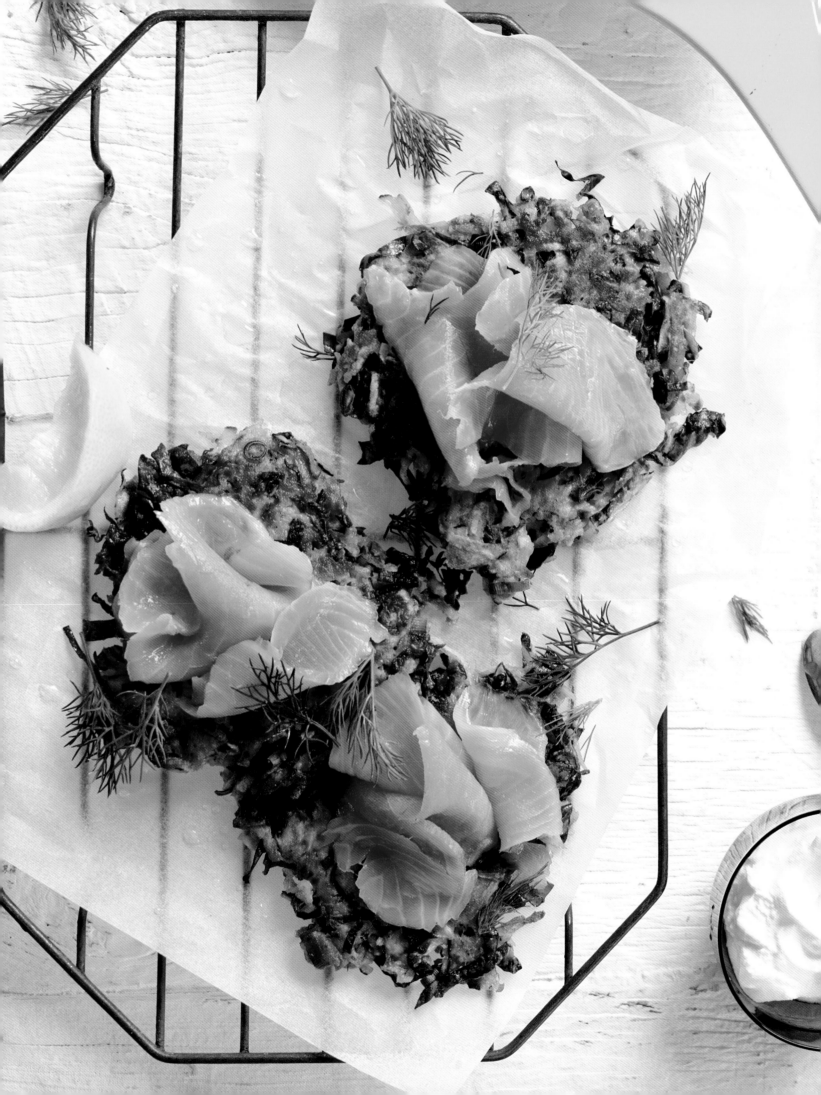

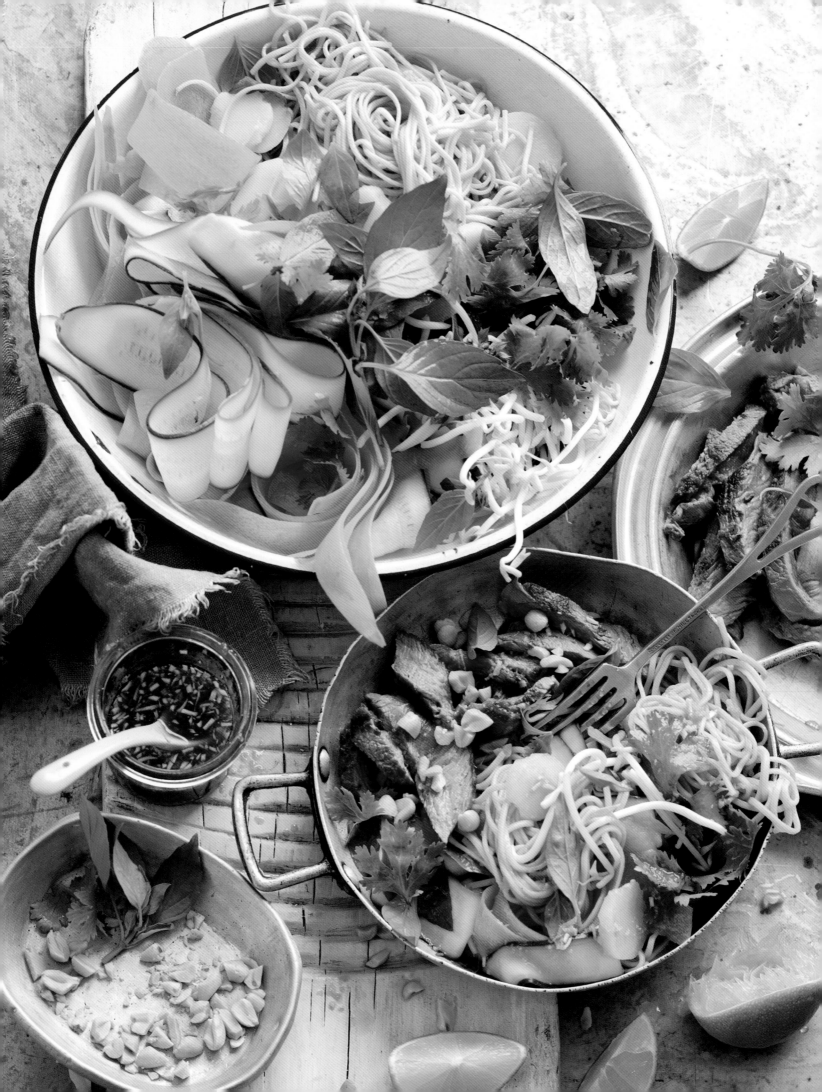

noodle salad with ginger-rubbed beef

PREP + COOK TIME 25 MINUTES ◆ **SERVES** 2

100g (3 ounces) soba noodles

200g (6½ ounces) beef rump steak, trimmed

2 teaspoons peanut oil

1 tablespoon finely grated fresh ginger

1 small zucchini (180g), cut into ribbons

1 small carrot (70g), cut into ribbons

60g (2 ounces) drained canned water chestnuts, sliced thinly

1 cup (80g) bean sprouts

½ cup fresh thai basil leaves

½ cup fresh coriander (cilantro) leaves

2 tablespoons lime juice

½ teaspoon sesame oil

1 clove garlic, crushed

3 teaspoons honey

1 teaspoon sodium-reduced soy sauce

2 tablespoons unsalted roasted peanuts, chopped coarsely

1 Cook noodles in a medium saucepan of boiling water, uncovered, for 4 minutes. Drain, rinse under cold water; drain well.

2 Rub steak with combined peanut oil and half the ginger. Season with pepper. Cook steak in a small heated non-stick frying pan for 2 minutes each side for medium or until cooked as desired. Stand covered for 5 minutes, then slice thinly.

3 Combine noodles, zucchini, carrot, chestnuts, sprouts, basil and coriander in a large bowl.

4 Combine remaining ginger, juice, sesame oil, garlic, honey and sauce in a screw-top jar; shake well. Pour over salad, toss gently to combine. Divide salad into serving bowls; top with steak, sprinkle with nuts.

TIPS You could also try this with ginger-rubbed chicken breast or firm tofu. Use a vegetable peeler or mandoline to cut vegetables into ribbons.

pork and veal lasagne with spinach

PREP + COOK TIME 1½ HOURS ◆ **SERVES** 2

1 tablespoon olive oil

200g (6½ ounces) mushrooms, chopped coarsely

1 medium brown onion (150g), chopped finely

1 clove garlic, crushed

200g (6½ ounces) lean minced (ground) pork and veal mixture (see tips)

400g (12½ ounces) canned no-added-salt diced tomatoes

1 tablespoon finely chopped fresh oregano

1 cup (250ml) skim milk

1¼ tablespoons cornflour (cornstarch)

250g (8 ounces) frozen chopped spinach, thawed

1 fresh lasagne sheet (50g), cut into thirds

¼ cup (25g) grated mozzarella

1 Preheat oven to 200°C/400°F. Lightly grease a 1-litre (4-cup) ovenproof dish.

2 Heat half the oil in a medium frying pan over high heat; cook mushrooms, stirring, for 5 minutes or until browned. Remove from pan.

3 Heat remaining oil in same pan over medium heat; cook onion and garlic, stirring, for 3 minutes or until onion is softened.

4 Increase heat to high, add mince to pan; cook, stirring, for 3 minutes or until browned. Return mushrooms to pan with tomatoes and oregano; simmer, covered, over low heat, for 10 minutes, stirring occasionally.

5 Meanwhile, combine milk and cornflour in a small saucepan; whisk until smooth. Cook, stirring, over medium heat, for 5 minutes or until mixture boils and thickens. Remove from heat.

6 Squeeze excess moisture from spinach.

7 Spoon a third of the mince mixture into prepared dish. Cover with one lasagne sheet. Spoon over another third of the mince mixture; top with spinach and another lasagne sheet. Spoon over remaining mince mixture; cover with lasagne sheet. Spoon over white sauce; sprinkle with cheese.

8 Place dish on an oven tray; bake for 45 minutes or until lasagne is tender and cheese is golden. Sprinkle with extra oregano leaves, if you like.

serving suggestion Serve with a leafy green salad.

TIPS This lasagne will freeze well, so make a double or triple batch in a larger ovenproof dish and freeze (once cooled) in individual airtight containers for up to 1 month. Some butcher's sell a pork and veal mixture, which is what we've used here. If it is not available, buy half the amount in pork mince and half the amount in veal mince.

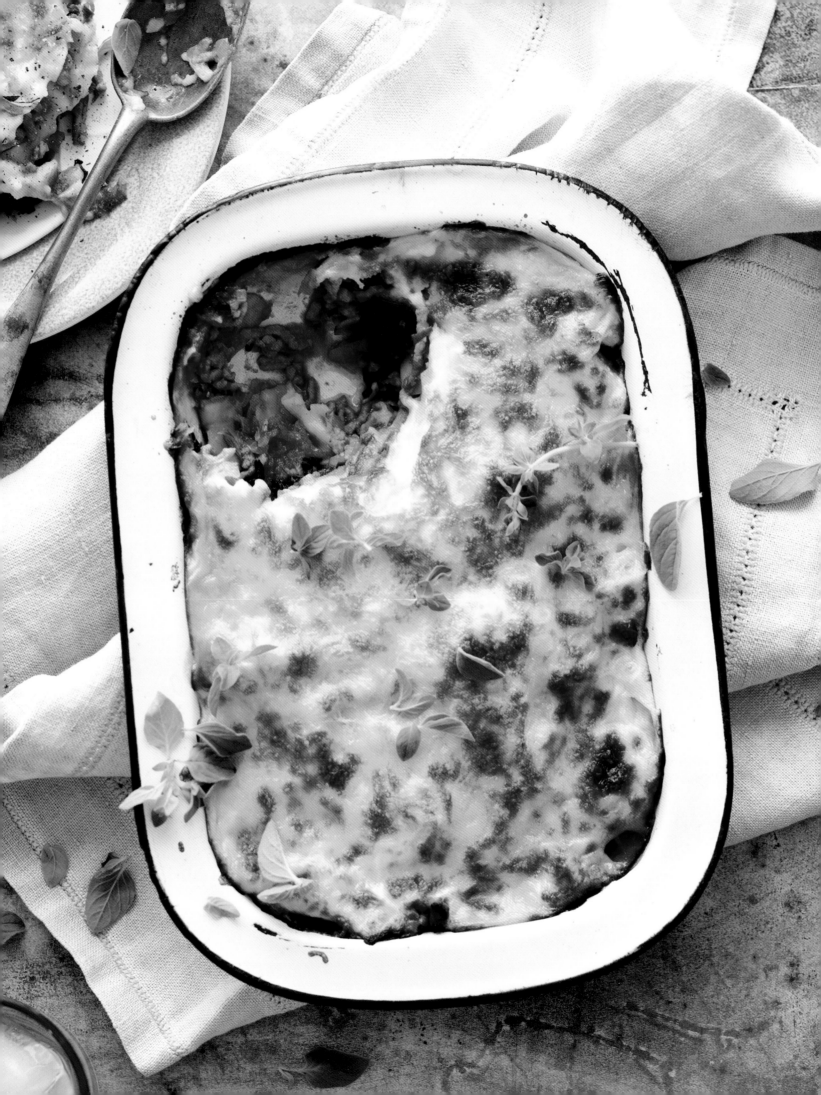

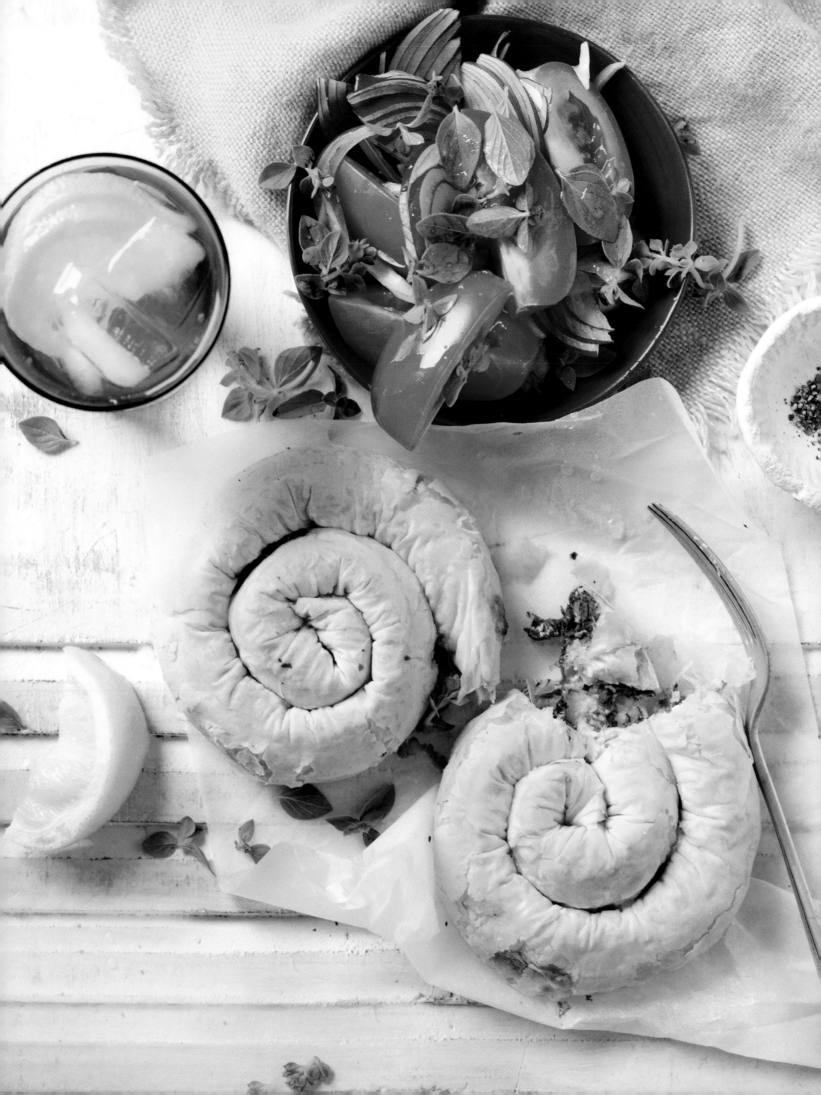

spinach and cheese snails

PREP + COOK TIME 50 MINUTES ◆ SERVES 2

6 medium silver beet leaves (swiss chard) (195g), trimmed, chopped roughly

cooking-oil spray

4 green onions (scallions), sliced thinly

1 clove garlic, crushed

½ cup (100g) low-fat low-salt cottage cheese

¼ cup finely-chopped fresh dill leaves

¼ cup finely chopped fresh flat-leaf parsley

1 egg yolk

4 sheets fillo pastry

TOMATO SALAD

2 medium roma (egg) tomatoes (150g), cut into wedges

1 small red onion (100g), sliced thinly

1 teaspoon olive oil

1 tablespoon fresh oregano leaves

1 Preheat oven to 180°C/350°F. Grease and line an oven tray with baking paper.

2 Cook silver beet in a large saucepan of boiling water for 5 minutes; drain, rinse under cold running water. Squeeze out excess moisture, place silver beet in a large bowl.

3 Spray a medium frying pan with oil; heat over low heat. Add onion and garlic to pan; cook, stirring occasionally, for 3 minutes or until soft.

4 Add onion mixture to silver beet with cheese, herbs and egg yolk; stir until well combined.

5 Spray one sheet of pastry with oil, top with another sheet. Spoon half the silver beet mixture along one long edge of the pastry and roll up tightly to form a sausage shape. Roll pastry to make a snail shape. Place on the oven tray. Repeat with remaining pastry and silver beet mixture.

6 Spray each snail lightly with oil; bake for 35 minutes or until pastry is crisp and golden.

7 Meanwhile, make tomato salad. Serve snails with salad.

TOMATO SALAD Combine ingredients in a medium bowl.

TIPS Make the filling a day ahead. The recipe is best baked just before serving.

italian white bean and cabbage soup

PREP + COOK TIME 1¼ HOURS (+ REFRIGERATION & STANDING) ◆ SERVES 2

1 cup (200g) dried cannellini beans

1 teaspoon olive oil

1 medium brown onion (150g), chopped coarsely

1 celery stalk (150g), chopped coarsely

2 cloves garlic, sliced thinly

1.5 litres (6 cups) salt-reduced vegetable stock

1 slice prosciutto (15g)

300g (9½ ounces) cabbage, shredded finely

3 teaspoons lemon juice

2 tablespoons fresh flat-leaf parsley leaves

1 Place beans in a medium bowl, cover with water; stand overnight. Rinse under cold water; drain.

2 Heat oil in a large saucepan over medium heat; cook onion, celery and garlic, stirring, for 5 minutes or until softened. Add stock and beans to the pan, bring to the boil; reduce heat, simmer, covered, for 50 minutes or until beans are tender.

3 Cook prosciutto in a non-stick frying pan, over high heat, for 1 minute each side or until crisp; break into shards.

4 Add cabbage to soup; simmer, covered, for 5 minutes or until just wilted. Stir in juice. Serve soup topped with prosciutto and parsley leaves.

TIPS Soak a large quantity of beans and boil until tender, store in the freezer in airtight bags so that you have beans on hand. You can use thinly sliced bacon or leftover roasted chicken instead of prosciutto. Add some finely shredded fresh sage leaves when frying the onion, if you like.

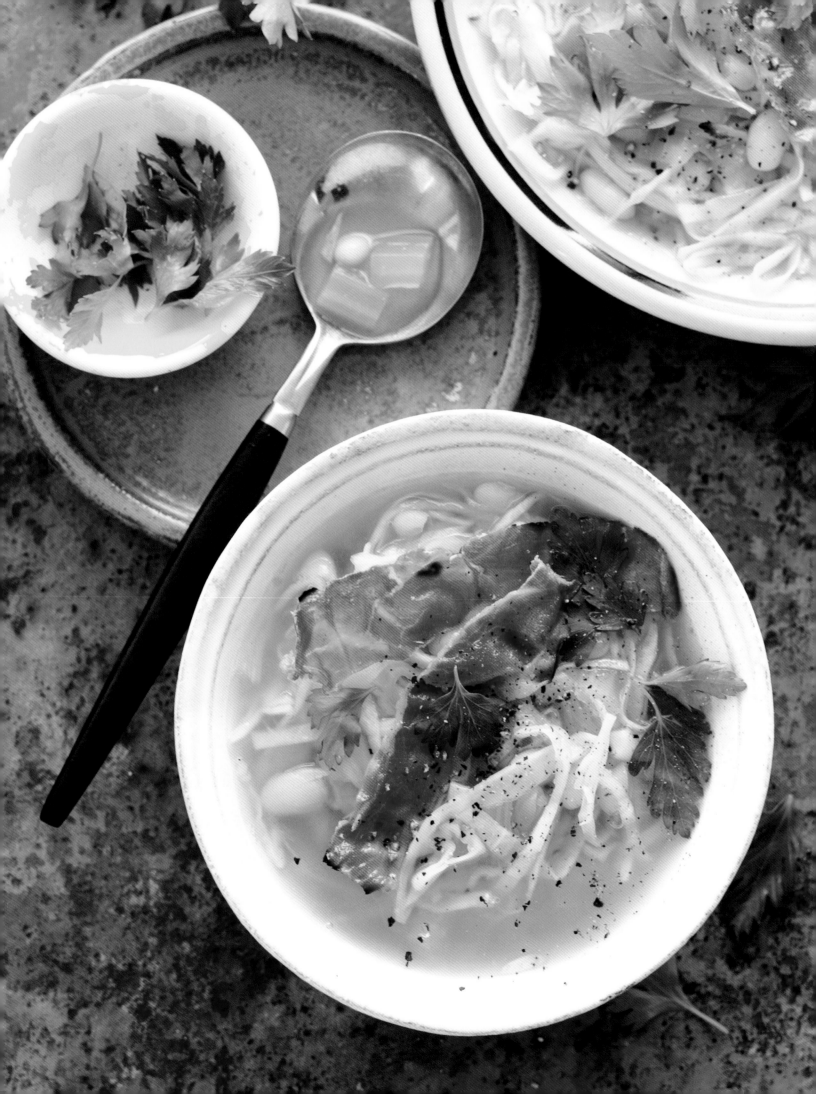

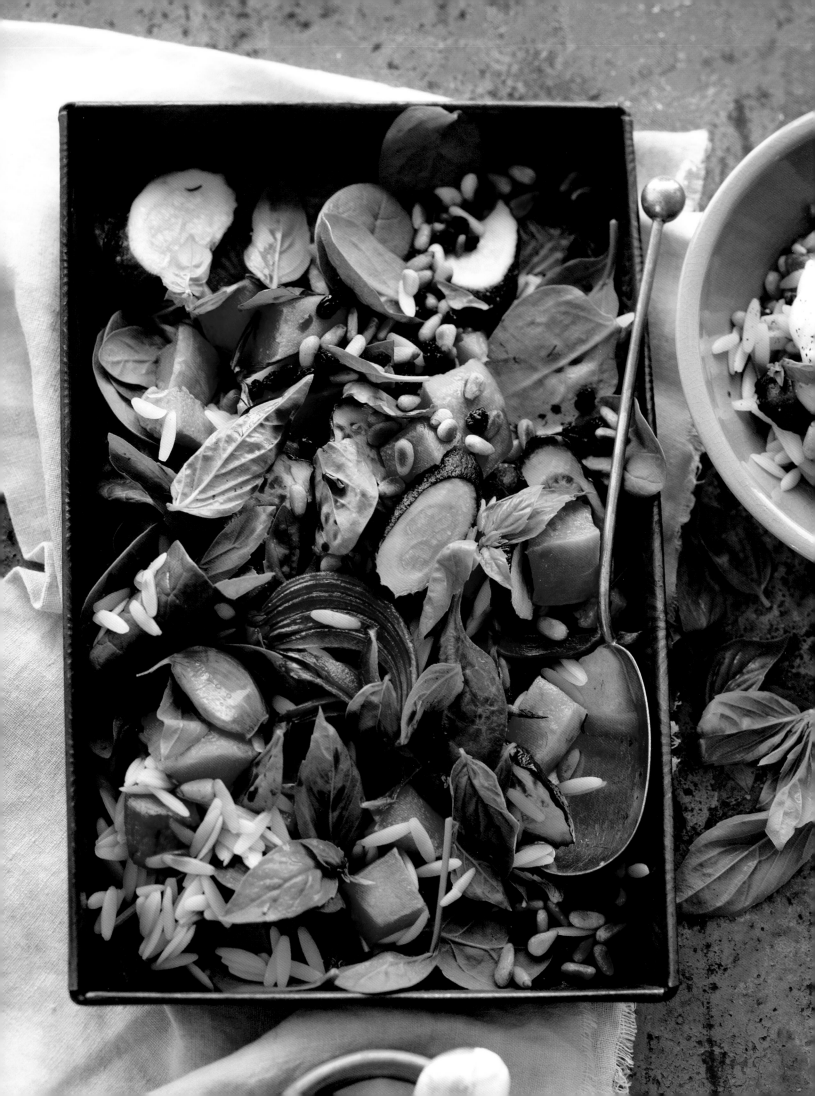

roast pumpkin and zucchini risoni salad

PREP + COOK TIME 45 MINUTES ◆ **SERVES** 2

250g (8 ounces) jap pumpkin, chopped coarsely

1 large zucchini (150g), chopped coarsely

1 small red onion (100g), cut into wedges

1 stalk fresh rosemary

9 small garlic cloves (35g), unpeeled

cooking-oil spray

⅓ cup (75g) risoni pasta

¼ cup (70g) low-fat plain yoghurt

1 tablespoon balsamic vinegar

1 cup loosely packed fresh basil leaves, torn

20g (¾ ounce) baby spinach leaves

1 tablespoon currants

2 tablespoons pine nuts, toasted

1 Preheat oven to 220°C/425°F.

2 Line a large roasting tray with baking paper. Combine pumpkin, zucchini, onion, rosemary and unpeeled garlic on the tray. Lightly spray with oil. Roast for 30 minutes or until tender and browned. Discard rosemary stalk.

3 Meanwhile, cook risoni in a large saucepan of boiling water until pasta is just tender. Drain, rinse under cold water, drain.

4 Peel garlic, place in a small bowl; mash with a fork. Add yoghurt and vinegar; stir to combine.

5 Combine the roasted vegetables in a large dish with risoni, basil, spinach, currants and pine nuts; stir through yoghurt mixture until just combined.

TIPS You can make this salad with other small pasta such as macaroni. Make the salad a day ahead but only dress it just before serving.

rocket, chicken and date salad

PREP + COOK TIME 40 MINUTES (+ COOLING) ◆ **SERVES** 2

300g (9½ ounces) chicken breast fillet, trimmed

3 cups (750ml) water

1 large orange (300g)

1½ tablespoons lemon juice

3 teaspoons fresh lemon thyme

2 teaspoons extra virgin olive oil

½ medium pomegranate (160g)

70g (2½ ounces) baby rocket leaves (arugula)

4 fresh dates (80g), seeded, quartered lengthways

12 dry roasted natural almonds (15g), chopped coarsely

1 Place chicken and the water in a small saucepan over high heat; bring to the boil. Reduce heat to low; simmer, uncovered, for 10 minutes. Remove from heat; cool for 20 minutes.

2 Meanwhile, using a zester, zest rind from half the orange in long thin strips. Peel orange, cut orange into segments, reserving 1½ tablespoons of juice.

3 To make dressing, combine juices, rind, thyme and oil in a small jug. Season with pepper.

4 Remove seeds from pomegranate; reserve.

5 Remove chicken from poaching liquid; shred chicken coarsely.

6 Arrange rocket on a large serving plate. Drizzle with a little dressing. Top with chicken, orange segments, dates, pomegranate seeds and nuts. Drizzle with remaining dressing.

TIPS If you don't have a zester, use a peeler to cut strips of orange rind, then cut the rind into thin strips. The chicken can be cooked a day ahead; cover, refrigerate.

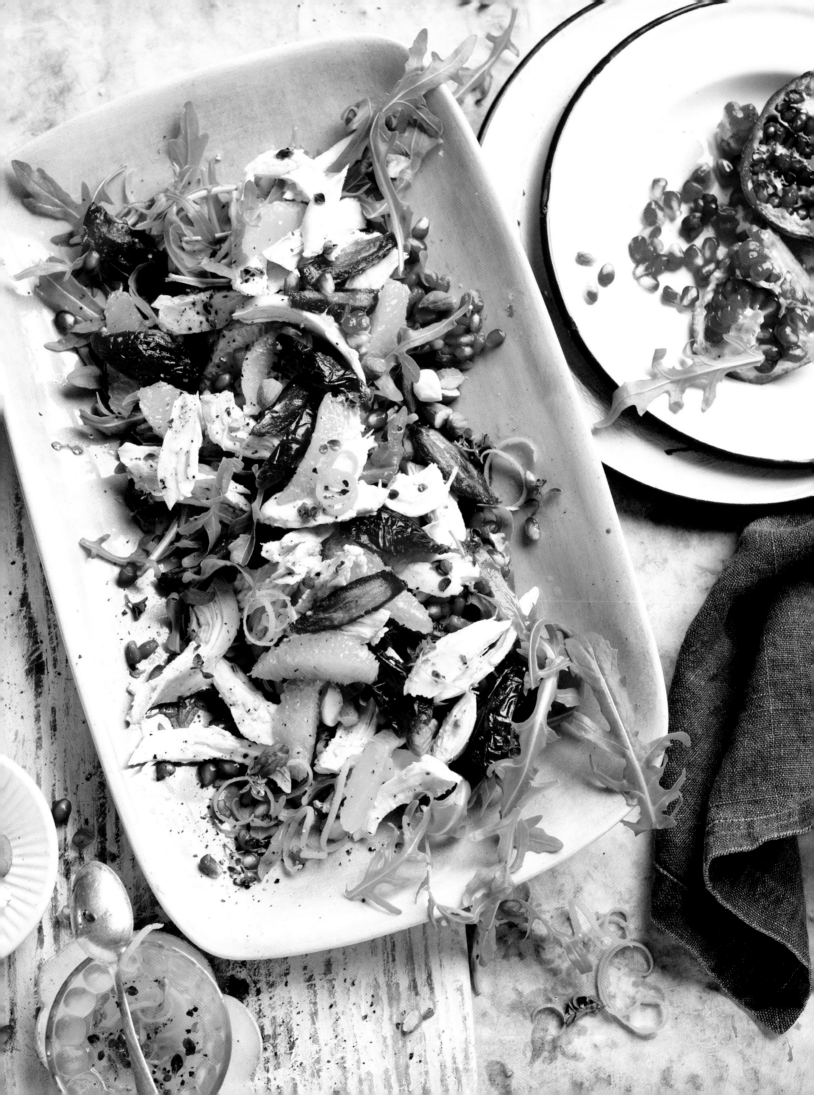

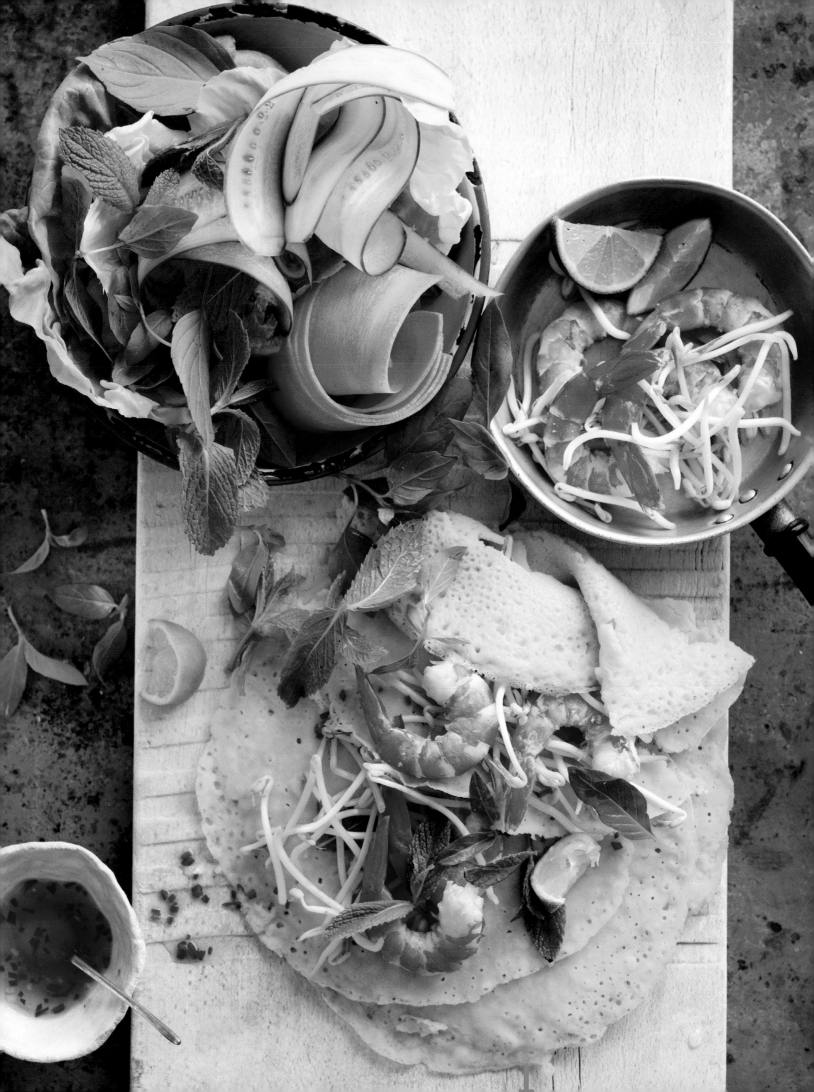

vietnamese pancakes with prawns

NUTRITIONAL COUNT PER SERVING

● 14.7g total fat   ● 23.5g protein

● 3.9g saturated fat   ● 6.5g fibre

● 1800kJ (430 cal)   ● 449mg sodium

● 47.1g carbohydrate   ● high GI

PREP + COOK TIME 30 MINUTES ◆ SERVES 4

8 cooked tiger prawns (shrimp) (280g)

½ cup (90g) rice flour

¼ teaspoon turmeric

2 tablespoons reduced-fat coconut milk

⅔ cup (160ml) water

1 egg

1 tablespoon olive oil

8 butter (boston) lettuce leaves (pulled from the centre of the lettuce)

1 lebanese cucumber (130g), sliced thinly

1 medium carrot (120g), sliced into ribbons

1 cup (80g) bean sprouts

½ bunch fresh mint leaves

½ bunch fresh thai basil leaves

CHILLI DIPPING SAUCE

1 tablespoon warm water

1 tablespoon lemon juice

2 teaspoons low-GI cane sugar

½ teaspoon fish sauce

½ clove garlic, crushed

1 fresh small red thai chilli (serrano), chopped finely

1 Make chilli dipping sauce.

2 Shell and devein prawns leaving tails intact.

3 Place rice flour and turmeric in a medium bowl. Add coconut milk, the water and egg; whisk until well combined and batter is smooth.

4 Heat 1 teaspoon of the oil in a large non-stick frying pan (base measurement 23cm/9-inches) over medium heat; pour a quarter of the batter into pan, swirl around base to form a thin pancake. Cook for 2 minutes or until batter has set.

5 Slide pancake onto a serving plate and repeat to make three more pancakes.

6 Serve pancakes with lettuce, prawns, cucumber, carrot, sprouts, herbs and chilli dipping sauce.

CHILLI DIPPING SAUCE Place the water, juice and sugar in a small bowl; stir until sugar has dissolved. Add remaining ingredients; stir to combine.

TIPS This traditional Vietnamese lunch is eaten by tearing off a piece of pancake and placing it inside a lettuce leaf, along with some herbs, sprouts, prawns and vegetables; it is then rolled up and dipped into a sauce. Use a vegetable peeler to slice thin ribbons from the cucumber and carrot.

- 23.6g total fat
- 3.7g saturated fat
- 2208kJ (527 cal)
- 29.6g carbohydrate
- 43.7g protein
- 18.1g fibre
- 220mg sodium
- medium GI

chermoula tuna, chickpea and broad bean salad

PREP + COOK TIME 30 MINUTES (+ REFRIGERATION) ◆ SERVES 2

200g (6½-ounce) piece tuna steak

1 cup (150g) frozen broad (fava) beans, thawed

150g (4½ ounces) green beans, trimmed, cut into thirds

420g (13½ ounce) canned no-added salt chickpeas (garbanzo beans), rinsed, drained

½ cup firmly packed fresh flat-leaf parsley leaves

1 medium lemon (140g), peeled, segmented

1 tablespoon lemon juice

1 tablespoon olive oil

CHERMOULA

½ small red onion (50g), chopped coarsely

1 clove garlic, peeled

1 cup firmly packed fresh coriander (cilantro), chopped roughly

1 cup firmly packed fresh flat-leaf parsley, chopped coarsely

1 teaspoon each ground cumin and smoked paprika

1 tablespoon olive oil

1 Make chermoula. Reserve three-quarters of the chermoula.

2 Place tuna in a shallow dish with remaining chermoula; toss to coat. Cover, refrigerate for 30 minutes.

3 Meanwhile, place broad beans in a heatproof bowl, cover with boiling water; stand for 2 minutes. Rinse under cold water; drain. Peel beans.

4 Boil, steam or microwave green beans until just tender; drain, rinse under cold water, drain.

5 Cook tuna on a heated oiled grill plate (or grill or barbecue) for 2 minutes each side or until slightly charred on the outside but still rare in the centre; cover, stand for 5 minutes. Cut tuna, across the grain, into slices.

6 Combine broad beans, green beans, chickpeas, parsley and lemon segments in a medium bowl with combined juice and oil. Serve tuna with salad and top with reserved chermoula.

CHERMOULA Blend or process ingredients until just combined.

TIPS Swap the tuna for salmon in this recipe. Purchase sashimi grade tuna for this recipe. If the chermoula ingredients aren't blending well, add 1 tablespoon water to the mixture.

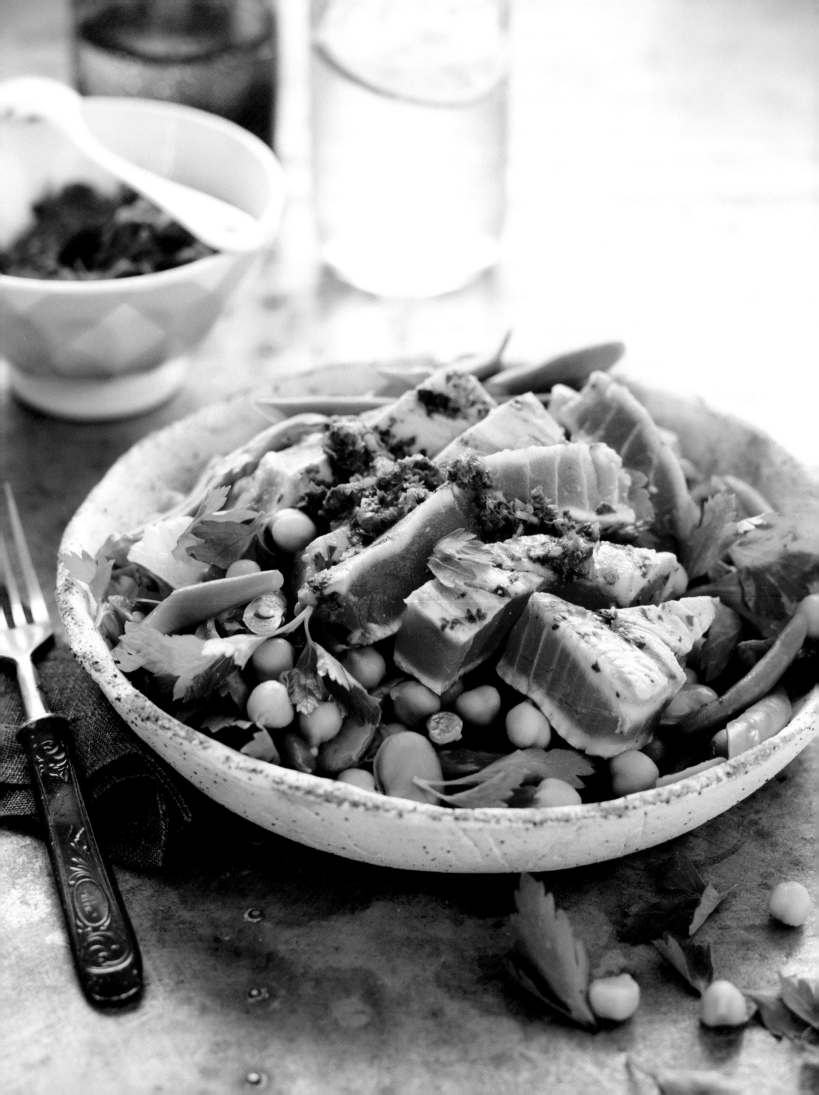

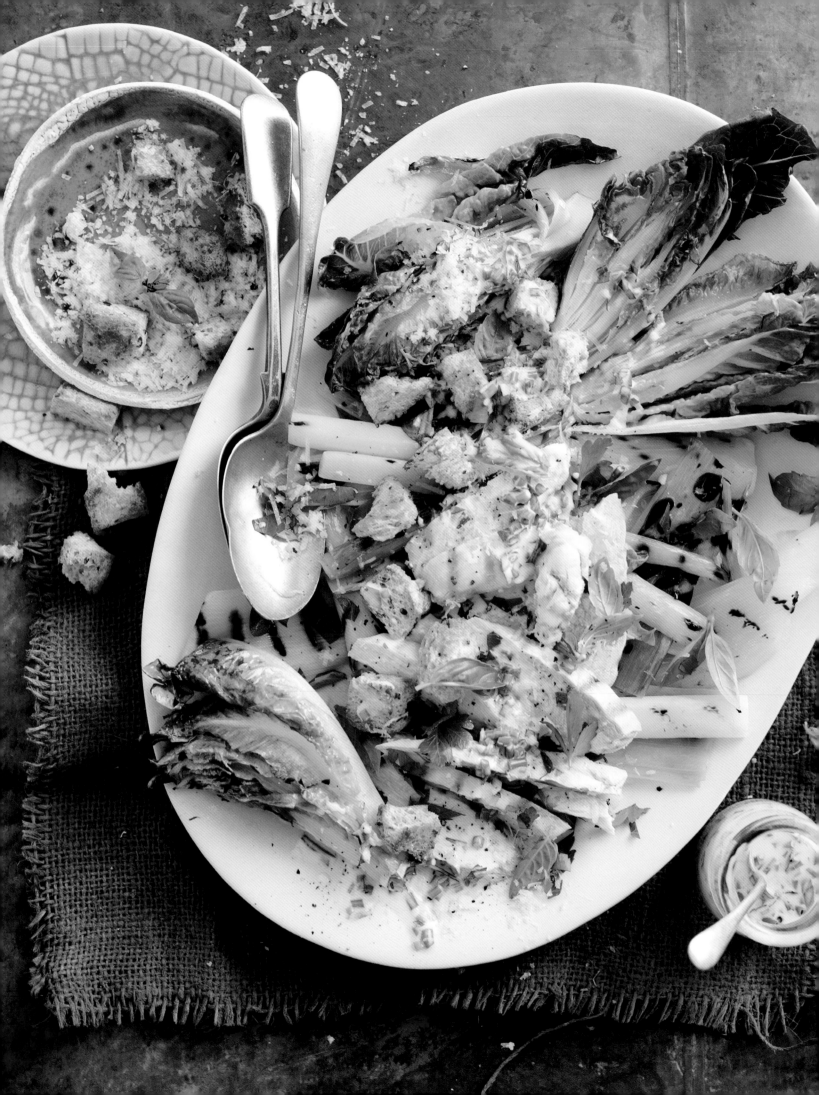

grilled chicken with warm cos lettuce salad

PREP + COOK TIME 1 HOUR ◆ SERVES 2

3 slices multigrain bread (100g), cut into 3cm (1¼-inch) cubes

rice bran oil spray

4 small leeks (800g), trimmed, halved lengthways

300g (9½ ounces) chicken breast fillet, trimmed

1 baby cos (romaine) lettuce (185g), trimmed, quartered lengthways

2 teaspoons finely grated lemon rind

1 tablespoon lemon juice

¼ cup coarsely chopped fresh basil leaves

¼ cup coarsely chopped fresh flat-leaf parsley

10g (½ ounce) shaved parmesan

BUTTERMILK DRESSING

¼ cup (60ml) buttermilk

3 teaspoons lemon juice

2 teaspoons chopped fresh tarragon

1 tablespoon chopped fresh chives

½ clove garlic, crushed

1 Preheat oven 200°C/400°F.

2 Place bread on a large oven tray in a single layer, spray with oil; bake for 10 minutes or until golden.

3 Cook leek in a medium pan of boiling water for 4 minutes or until just tender; drain.

4 Heat a lightly oiled grill plate (or grill or barbecue) over high heat; cook chicken for 3 minutes each side or until golden brown. Place chicken on an oven tray; cover with foil. Transfer to oven; bake for 15 minutes or until just cooked through. Rest for 10 minutes, then slice thickly.

5 Meanwhile, spray leeks and lettuce with oil; cook leeks on the grill plate for 3 minutes or until browned and the lettuce for 1 minute or until browned lightly, turning halfway through cooking time.

6 Make buttermilk dressing.

7 Combine chicken in a bowl with rind, juice, basil and parsley.

8 To serve, top lettuce wedges with leeks and chicken mixture; sprinkle with croûtons and parmesan and drizzle with buttermilk dressing. Sprinkle with extra basil and parsley leaves, if you like.

BUTTERMILK DRESSING Combine ingredients in a small jug; season with pepper to taste.

TIP You can substitute the leeks with green onions (scallions) or asparagus.

lime and coriander beef salad

PREP + COOK TIME 35 MINUTES ◆ SERVES 2

80g (2½ ounces) udon noodles

200g (6½ ounces) beef rump steak, trimmed

1 cup loosely packed fresh coriander leaves (cilantro)

1 tablespoon finely grated lime rind

1 lebanese cucumber (130g), cut into ribbons

2 medium tomatoes (300g), chopped coarsely

⅓ cup loosely packed fresh mint leaves

3 green onions (scallions), sliced thinly

100g (3 ounces) snow peas, sliced thinly

50g (1½ ounce) snow pea sprouts

¼ cup (35g) coarsely chopped unsalted roasted cashews

LIME DRESSING

2 tablespoons lime juice

1 teaspoon fish sauce

2 teaspoons finely chopped palm sugar

1 fresh long red chilli, chopped finely

1 Place noodles in a medium heatproof bowl, cover with boiling water; stand for 5 minutes or until just tender, drain. Refresh under cold water; drain.

2 Meanwhile, make dressing.

3 Cook beef on a heated oiled grill plate (or grill or barbecue) for 1 minute each side or until cooked as desired. Cover, rest for 5 minutes.

4 Meanwhile, finely chop half the coriander. Combine chopped coriander and rind on a plate. Coat beef in coriander mixture; slice beef thinly.

5 Add remaining coriander, cucumber, tomato, mint, onion, snow peas, sprouts, dressing and beef to noodles; toss gently to combine. Sprinkle with nuts to serve.

LIME DRESSING Combine ingredients in a screw-top jar; shake to combine.

TIP Use a vegetable peeler to cut cucumber into ribbons.

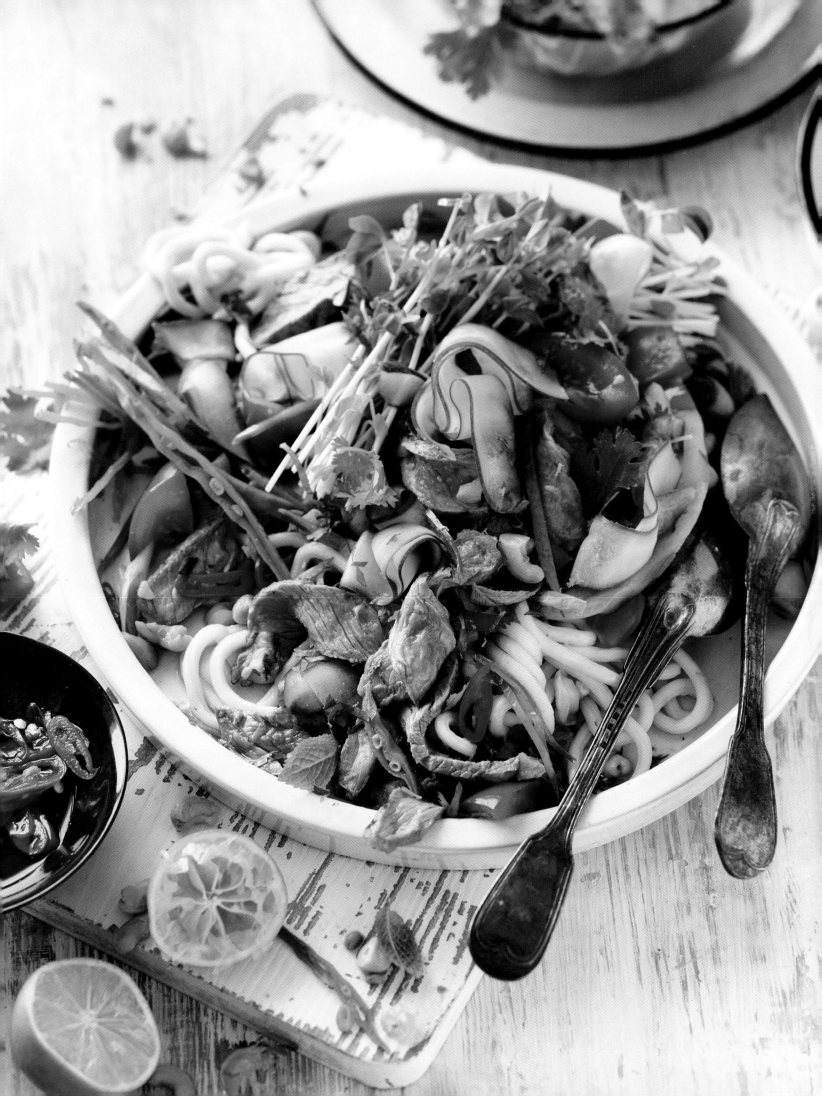

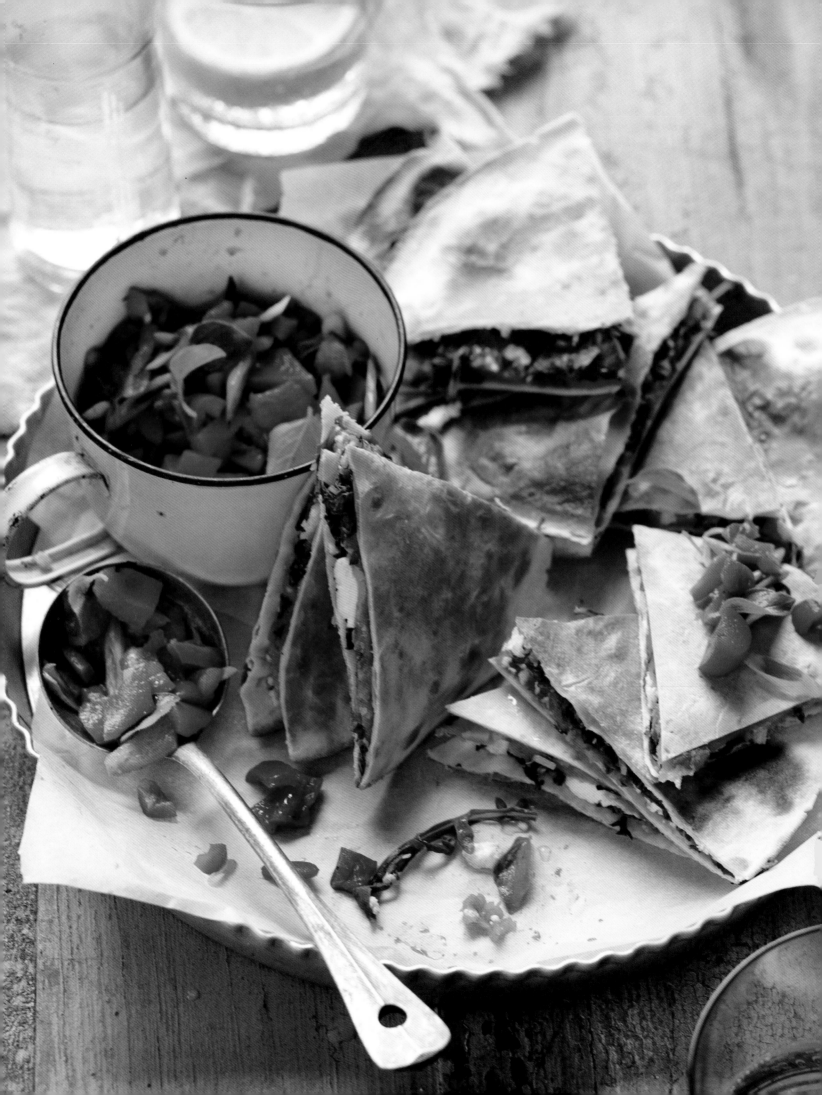

NUTRITIONAL COUNT PER SERVING

● 9g total fat
● 2.3g saturated fat
● 1715kJ (410 cal)
● 60.8g carbohydrate
● 15.2g protein
● 12.2g fibre
● 256mg sodium
● low GI

pumpkin, ricotta and rocket quesadillas

PREP + COOK TIME 1¼ HOURS ◆ SERVES 2

500g (1 pound) butternut pumpkin, peeled, chopped into 4cm (1½-inch) pieces

rice bran oil spray

2 teaspoons each ground cumin and coriander

2 teaspoons coarsely chopped fresh oregano

4 white corn tortillas

50g (1½ ounces) baby rocket leaves (arugula)

⅓ cup (80g) low-fat ricotta

ROASTED CAPSICUM SALSA

1 small red capsicum (bell pepper) (150g), quartered, seeded

1 green onion (scallion), sliced thinly

2 teaspoons coarsely chopped fresh oregano

¼ teaspoon smoked paprika

1 teaspoon balsamic vinegar

1 Preheat oven 200°C/400°F. Line a large baking tray with baking paper.

2 Place pumpkin on baking tray, spray with oil then sprinkle with cumin and coriander; cover with foil. Bake for 45 minutes or until tender. Cool slightly, mash with a fork. Stir in oregano; cool.

3 Meanwhile make roasted capsicum salsa.

4 Spread half the pumpkin mixture over 1 tortilla; top with half the rocket. Spread another tortilla with half the ricotta. Sandwich tortillas and spray both sides with oil spray.

5 Heat a medium non-stick frying pan over medium heat; cook tortillas for 2 minutes each side or until browned and heated through. Repeat with remaining ingredients.

6 Cut quesadillas into wedges; serve with salsa.

ROASTED CAPSICUM SALSA Preheat grill (broiler) to high. Place capsicum, skin-side up, on a large oven tray. Grill for 10 minutes or until skin is blackened. Cover tray with foil. Stand for 10 minutes to cool. Peel and discard skin; roughly chop capsicum. Combine capsicum in a small bowl with remaining ingredients. Season with black pepper to taste.

TIP You can use 120g (4 ounces) drained char-grilled capsicum, if you like.

spiced vegetable, chickpea and ricotta salad

PREP + COOK TIME 1 HOUR ◆ **SERVES** 2

200g (6½ ounces) baby carrots, trimmed

1 small kumara (orange sweet potato) (250g), cut into 2cm (¾-inch) wedges

½ small red onion (50g) cut into wedges

½ medium red capsicum (bell pepper) (175g), sliced thickly

½ x 400g (12½ ounces) canned chickpeas (garbanzo beans), rinsed, drained

1 tablespoon rice bran oil

1 teaspoon each ground cumin and coriander

150g (4 ounce) fresh ricotta

large pinch each dried chilli flakes and oregano

150g (4 ounces) vine-ripened baby cherry truss tomatoes

2 tablespoons roughly chopped walnuts

2 tablespoons fresh flat-leaf parsley leaves, torn

1 Preheat oven to 200°C/400°F. Line an oven tray with baking paper.

2 Place carrot, kumara, onion, capsicum and chickpeas on tray. Drizzle with half the oil and sprinkle with cumin and coriander. Toss gently to combine.

3 Place ricotta on tray alongside vegetables. Drizzle with remaining oil; sprinkle with chilli and oregano. Bake ricotta and vegetables for 40 minutes or until vegetables are tender, adding tomatoes to tray for the last 10 minutes of cooking time.

4 Serve ricotta with vegetables sprinkled with nuts and parsley.

TIP You can use heirloom baby carrots, which would add great colour to this dish.

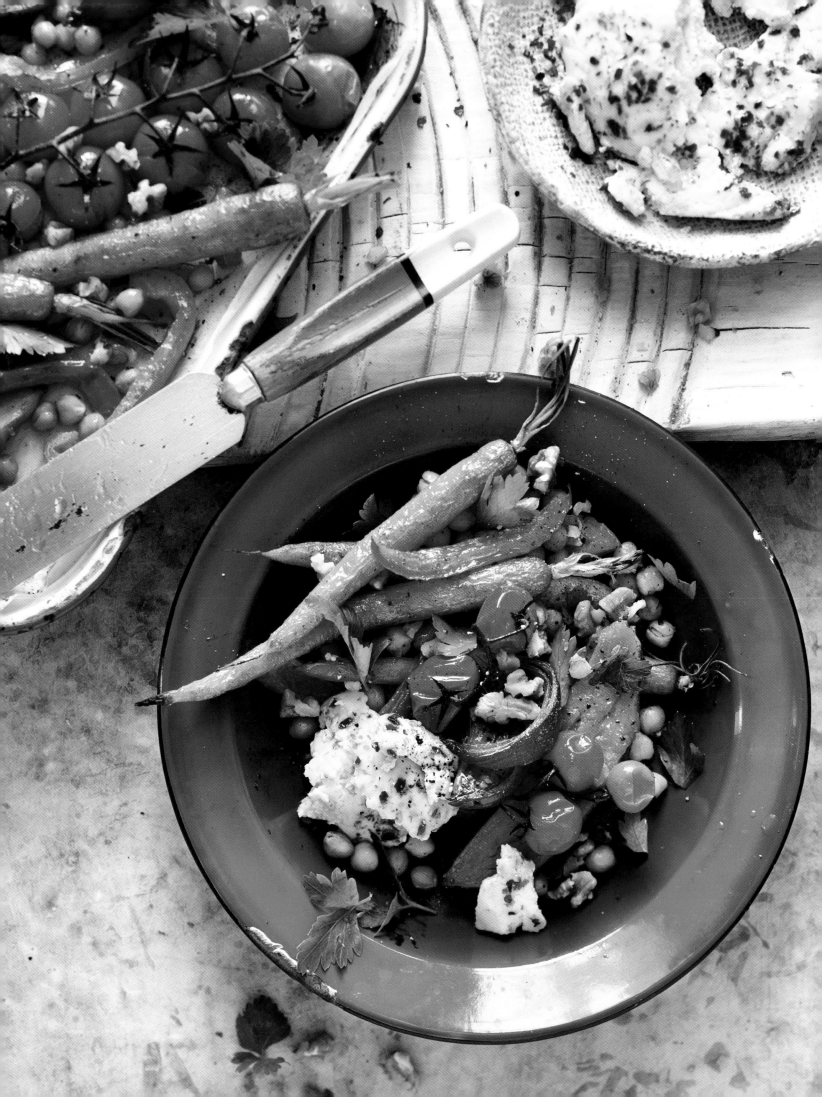

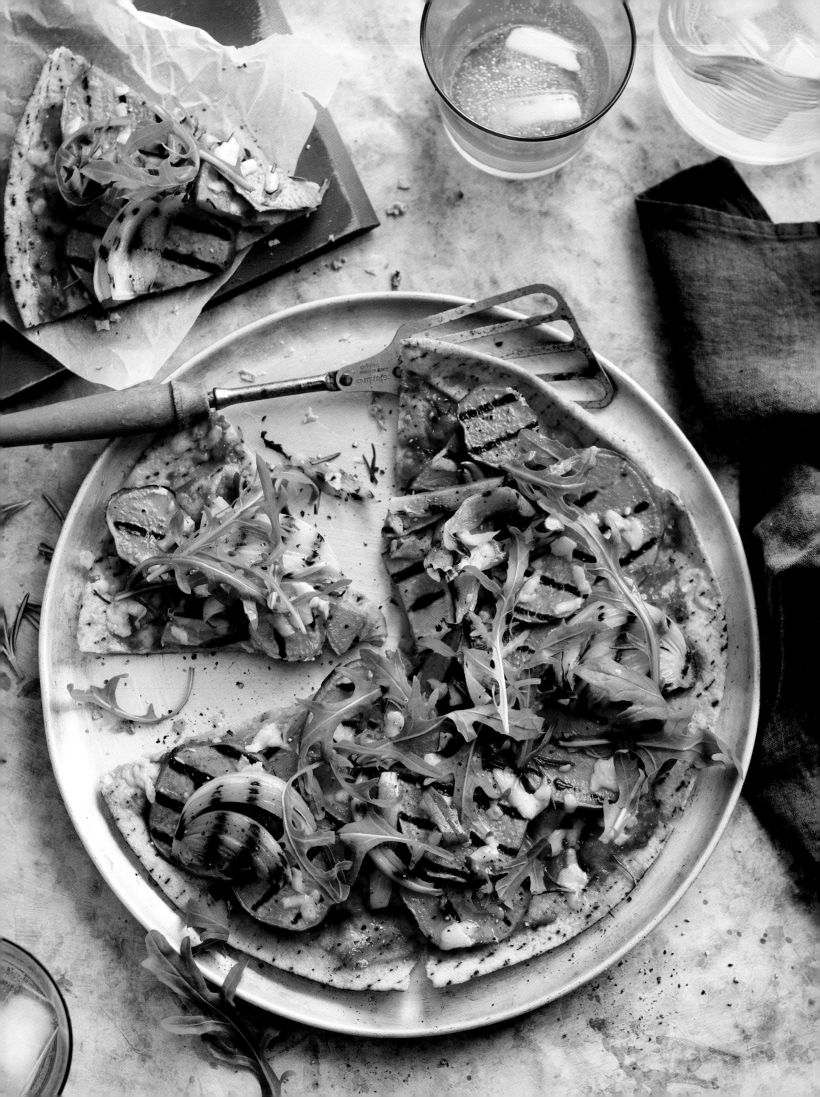

NUTRITIONAL COUNT PER SERVING

● 5.2g total fat   ● 12g protein
● 2.6g saturated fat   ● 6.6g fibre
● 1198kJ (286 cal)   ● 420mg sodium
● 44.3g carbohydrate   ● medium GI

kumara and onion pizza

PREP + COOK TIME 30 MINUTES ◆ SERVES 2

1 small kumara (orange sweet potato) (250g), unpeeled, sliced thinly

½ small brown onion (40g), cut into thin wedges

1 large wholemeal pitta bread (100g)

2 tablespoons salt-reduced tomato pasta sauce

1½ teaspoons finely chopped fresh rosemary

¼ cup (30g) coarsely grated low-fat vintage cheddar

20g (¾ ounce) baby rocket leaves (arugula)

1 Preheat oven to 220°C/425°F. Line an oven tray with baking paper.

2 Cook kumara and onion on a heated oiled grill plate (or grill or barbecue) until browned both sides and tender.

3 Place bread on oven tray; spread with sauce. Layer with vegetables and sprinkle with rosemary then cheese. Bake for 8 minutes or until base is crisp and cheese has melted. Serve topped with rocket.

broad bean, apple & walnut open sandwich

PREP + COOK TIME 20 MINUTES ◆ SERVES 2

1 cup (150g) frozen broad beans, thawed

1 teaspoon finely grated lemon rind

1 tablespoon lemon juice

1 tablespoon coarsely chopped fresh dill

1 tablespoon coarsely chopped fresh mint

2 trimmed celery stalks (200g), sliced thinly

½ small red apple (65g), sliced thinly

¼ cup (25g) coarsely chopped walnuts

2 thick slices multigrain sourdough bread (140g), toasted

2 tablespoons cashew nut spread

4 baby cos (romaine) lettuce leaves (20g)

5g (¼ ounce) micro watercress

1 Place broad beans in a large heatproof bowl, cover with boiling water; stand for 3 minutes. Rinse under cold water; drain, then peel.

2 Combine beans, rind, juice, dill, mint, celery, apple and walnuts in a large bowl. Season with pepper to taste.

3 Spread bread slices with half the cashew spread each. Top each with a lettuce leaf and half of the bean mixture.

4 Sprinkle with watercress and top with extra lemon rind, if you like.

TIP Cashew spread can be found in the health food aisle of the supermarket or at health food stores.

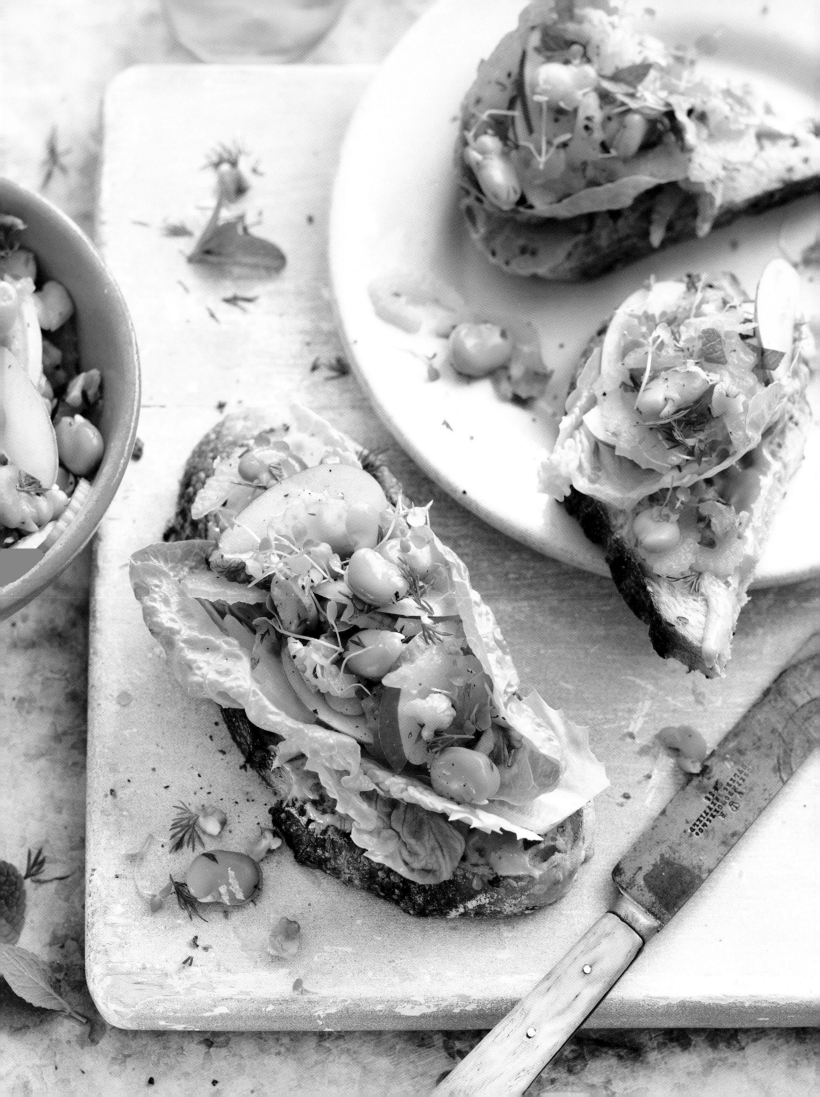

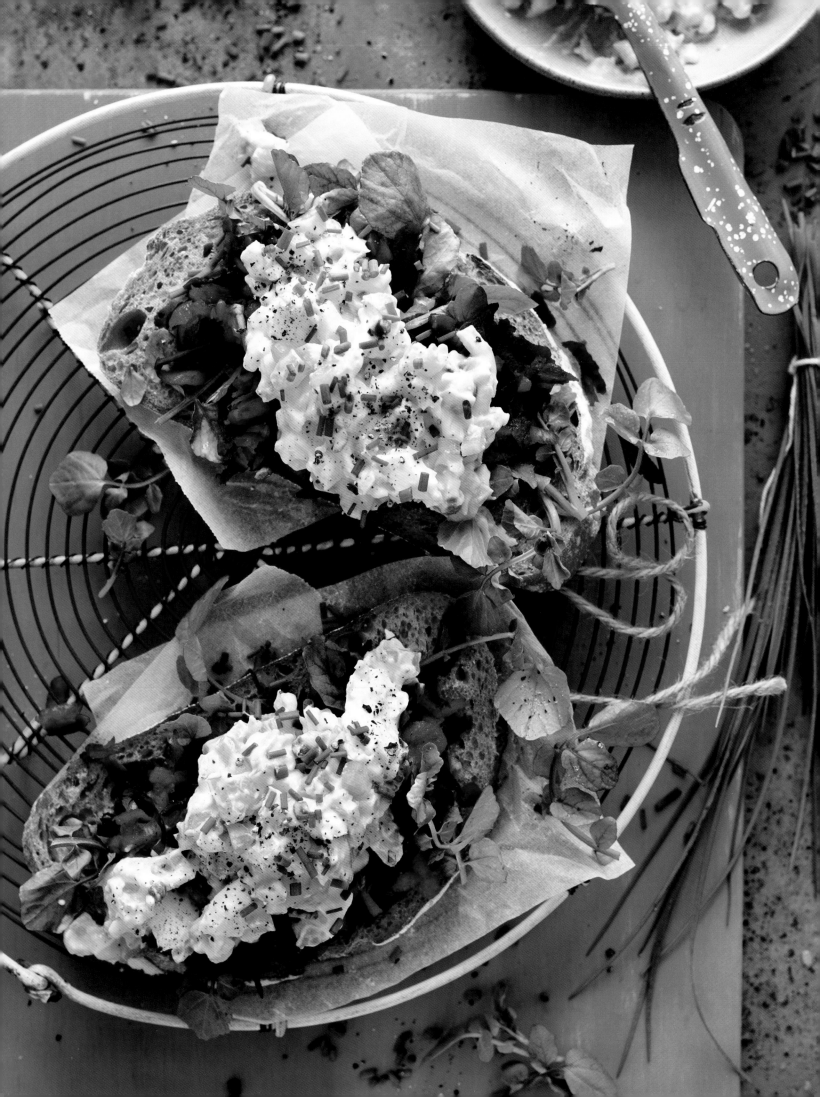

creamy egg salad open sandwich

PREP + COOK TIME 15 MINUTES ◆ **SERVES** 2

3 small eggs, at room temperature

2 tablespoons low-fat greek yoghurt

1 tablespoon low-fat mayonnaise

2 teaspoons dijon mustard

2 teaspoons rice bran oil

2 teaspoons baby capers, rinsed, drained, chopped

1 trimmed stalk celery (100g), chopped finely

1 small beetroot (beet) (100g), peeled, grated coarsely

2 red radishes (70g), grated coarsely

2 thin slices rye bread (90g), toasted

1 cup loosely packed watercress leaves (120g)

1 tablespoon finely chopped fresh chives

1 Place eggs in a small saucepan; cover with cold water, cover pan with a lid. Bring water to the boil, then remove lid. Boil for 5 minutes, then remove from heat; drain. When cool enough to handle, shell eggs.

2 Roughly mash eggs in a medium bowl with yoghurt, mayonnaise, mustard, oil, capers and celery.

3 Combine beetroot and radish in a small bowl.

4 Top each bread slice with half the watercress, beetroot and radish mixture, then egg mixture. Sprinkle with chives; season with pepper to taste.

TIP You can make the egg mixture a day ahead. Store in an airtight container in the fridge and assemble sandwiches just before serving.

roasted brussels sprouts & lentil salad

PREP + COOK TIME 1½ HOURS ◆ SERVES 2

¾ cup (150g) dried french-style green lentils

1½ cups (375ml) water

8 brussels sprouts, trimmed, halved

olive-oil spray

2 tablespoons slivered almonds, toasted

¼ cup fresh mint leaves

2 tablespoons low-fat balsamic vinaigrette

2 tablespoons shaved parmesan

1 Place lentils and the water in a small saucepan, bring to the boil over high heat. Reduce heat to low; simmer, covered, for 45 minutes or until lentils are tender. Drain.

2 Preheat oven to 200°C/400°F.

3 Cook sprouts in a small saucepan of boiling water, uncovered, for 3 minutes; drain. Line an oven tray with baking paper. Spread sprouts on tray; spray with oil. Transfer to oven; roast for 20 minutes or until golden.

4 Place lentils, sprouts, nuts, mint, vinaigrette and parmesan in a bowl; season with pepper to taste. Toss to combine.

TIPS This is a great side for grilled chicken or fish. If brussels sprouts aren't available use chopped cabbage.

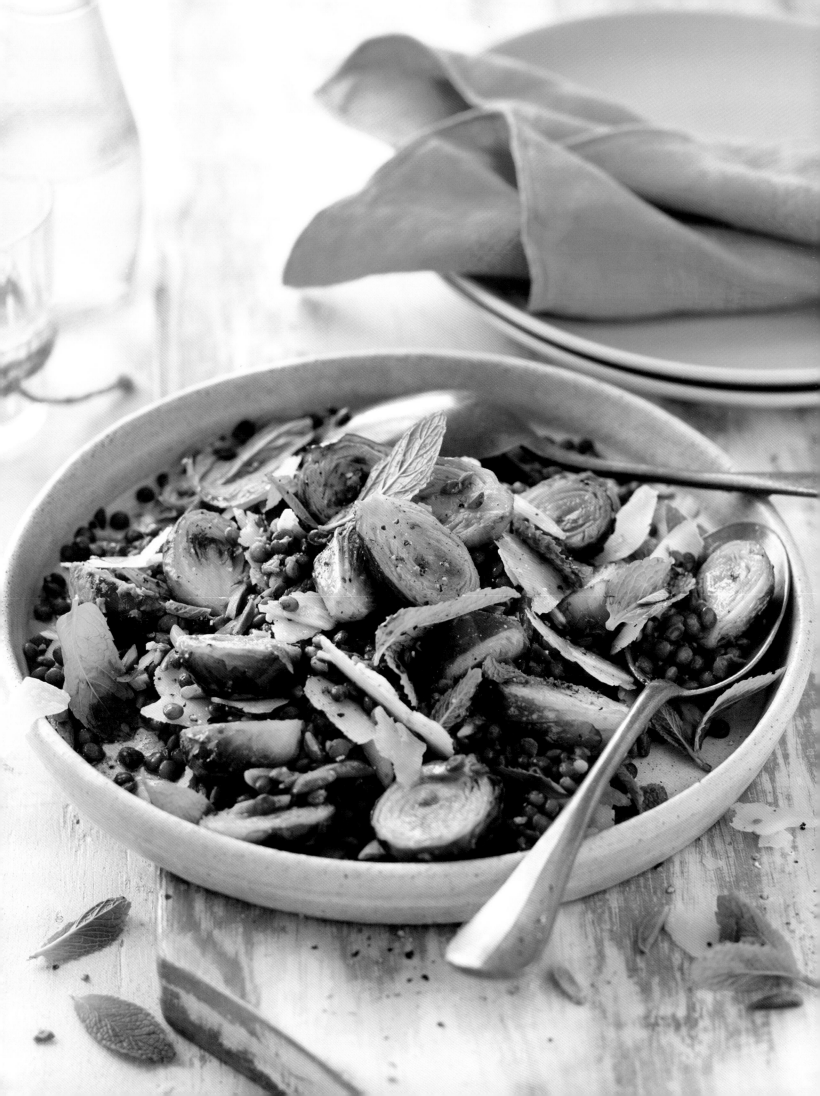

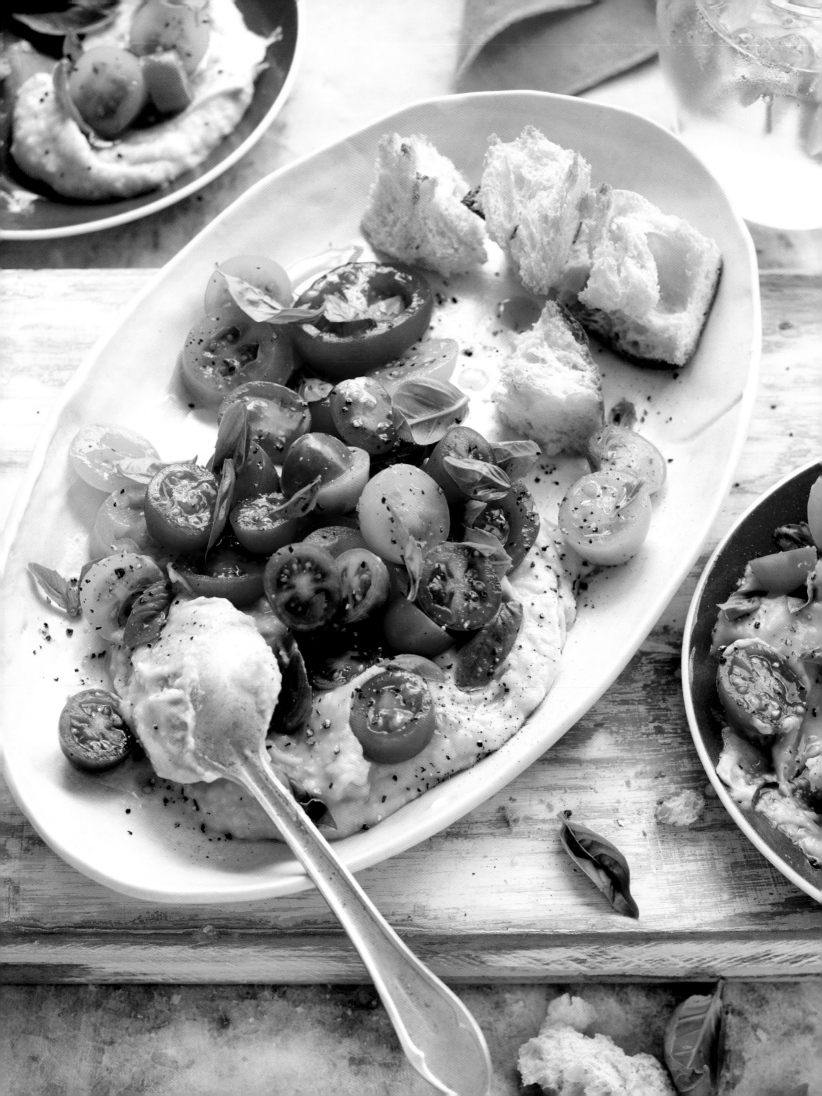

NUTRITIONAL COUNT PER SERVING

● 6.2g total fat   ● 9.9g protein

● 0.9g saturated fat   ● 7.6g fibre

● 1013kJ (242 cal)   ● 406mg sodium

● 32.2g carbohydrate   ● low GI

tomato & white bean puree salad

PREP + COOK TIME 25 MINUTES ◆ **SERVES** 2

80g (2½ ounce) ciabatta bread, torn

200g (12 ½ ounces) canned cannellini beans, rinsed, drained

1 garlic clove, crushed

2 teaspoons lemon juice

2 teaspoons rice bran oil

200g (6 ½ ounces) medley tomatoes, sliced

3 teaspoons red wine vinegar

2 tablespoons small fresh basil leaves

1 Preheat grill (broiler) to high. Place bread on an oven tray; grill for 1 minute or until browned lightly.

2 Blend or process beans, garlic, juice and oil until mixture is smooth. Season with pepper to taste.

3 Combine tomato, vinegar and two-thirds of the basil in a small bowl; toss gently to combine. Serve bean mixture topped with tomato salad and bread; sprinkle with remaining basil.

TIP Depending on the brand of beans used, you may need to add 1 tablespoon water to reach the desired consistency.

NUTRITIONAL COUNT PER SERVING

- 10.5g total fat
- 2.9g saturated fat
- 1903kJ (455 cal)
- 28.8g carbohydrate
- 58.1g protein
- 5g fibre
- 128mg sodium
- medium GI

ginger and chilli chicken rice paper rolls

PREP TIME 20 MINUTES ◆ **SERVES** 2

50g (1½ ounces) rice vermicelli noodles

2 tablespoons finely grated ginger

1 teaspoon peanut oil

2 teaspoons lime juice

2 teaspoons chinese cooking wine

2 skinless cooked chicken breast fillets (400g), sliced thickly

6 x 22cm (9-inch) rice paper rounds

12 fresh coriander (cilantro) sprigs

1 small carrot (70g), grated coarsely

2 green onions (scallions), halved lengthways, cut into matchsticks

½ small red capsicum (bell pepper) (150g), cut into matchsticks

½ lebanese cucumber (65g), cut into matchsticks

½ long red chilli, seeded, sliced thinly

⅓ cup bean sprouts (25g)

1 Place noodles in a large heatproof bowl; cover with boiling water, separate noodles with a fork. Stand until tender; drain.

2 Place ginger in a fine sieve over a medium bowl; press down firmly on ginger to remove juice; discard pulp. Add oil, lime juice and cooking wine to ginger juice. Gently toss chicken and noodles through the ginger mixture.

3 Dip one rice paper round into a bowl of warm water until soft. Lift sheet from water; place on a clean tea towel. Place two coriander sprigs on the rice paper, top with one-sixth of the noodle mixture, carrot, onion, capsicum, cucumber, chilli and sprouts. Fold rice sheet over filling, then fold in both sides. Continue rolling to enclose filling, repeat with remaining ingredients to make a total of 6 rolls. Serve with a wedge of lime, if you like.

TIPS Rice paper rolls can be prepared up to 1 day ahead of serving. Cover with damp paper towel and plastic wrap until ready to serve. You can use poached chicken breast or the breast from a barbecued or roasted chicken.

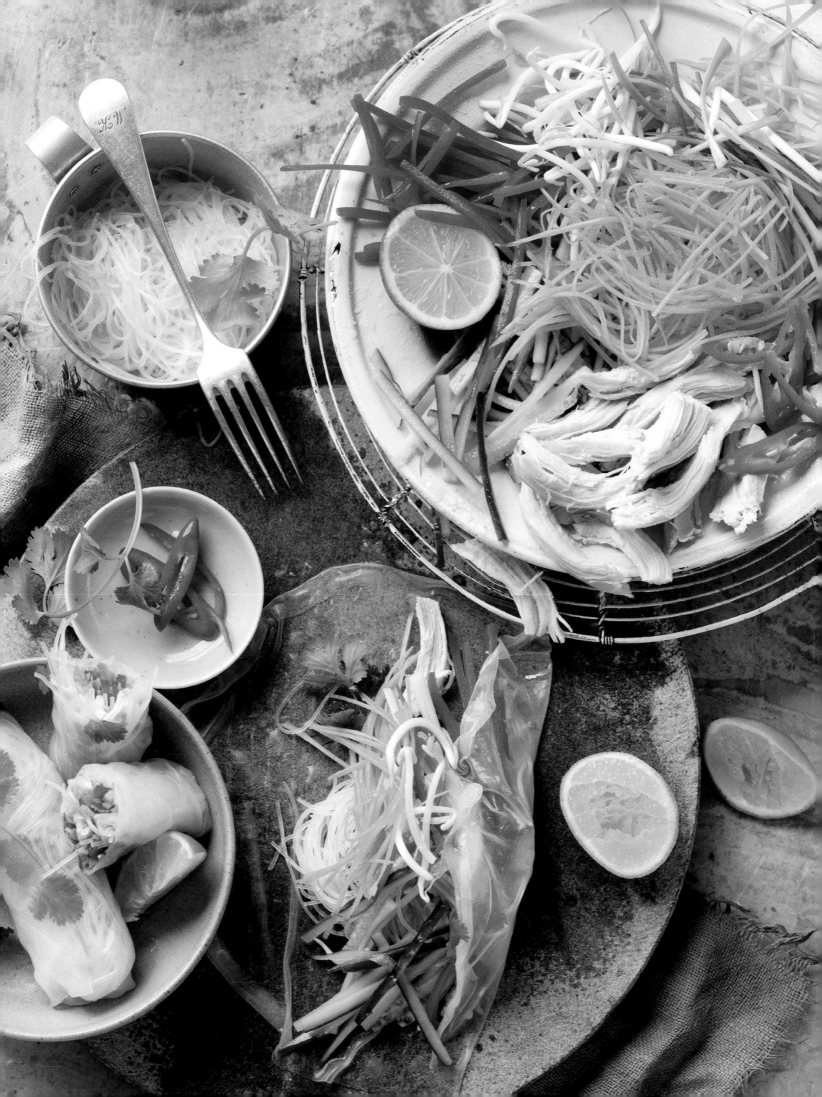

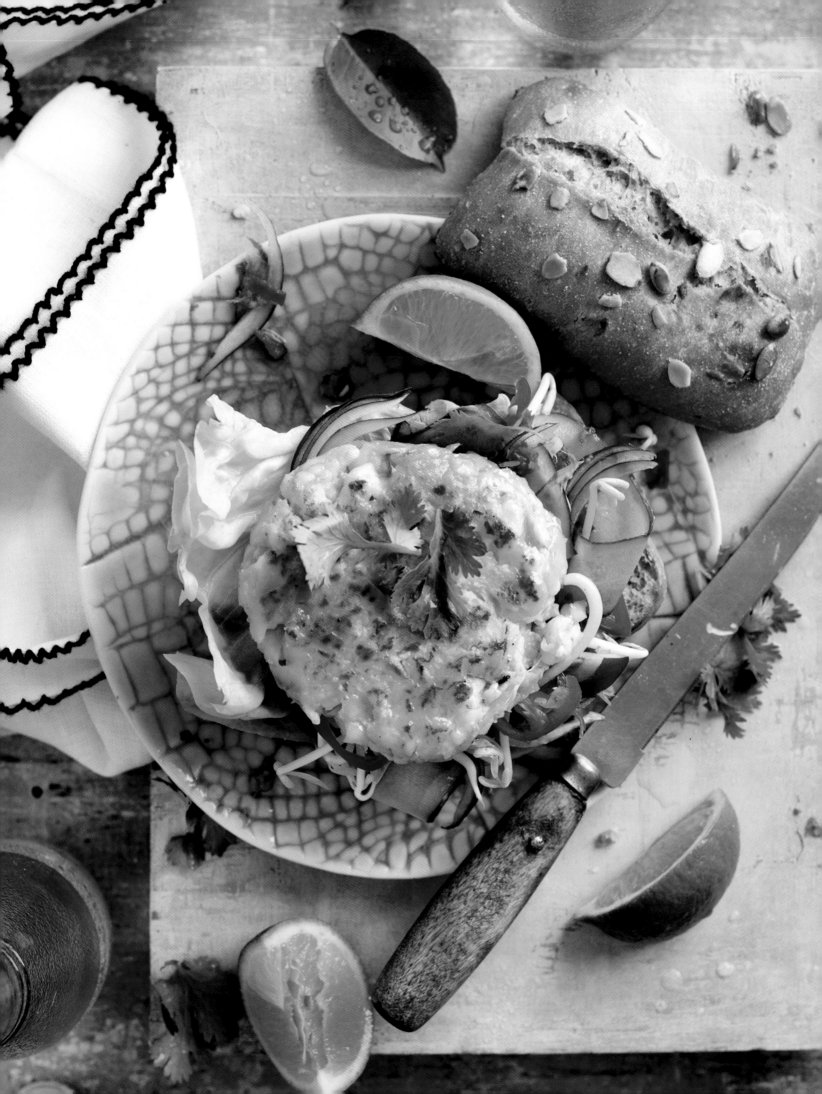

thai prawn burgers

PREP + COOK TIME 20 MINUTES (+ REFRIGERATION) ◆ **SERVES** 2

1 clove garlic

2 coriander roots (cilantro), with 1cm (½-inch) stem attached

2 teaspoons coarsely chopped fresh ginger

2 kaffir lime leaves, shredded

2 fresh long red chillies, sliced thinly

8 uncooked, peeled small king prawns (shrimp) (100g), chopped finely

1 small potato (120g), coarsely grated

1 tablespoon rice bran oil

3 teaspoons lime juice

2 small wholemeal bread rolls (85g), split in half crossways

4 medium butter lettuce leaves

½ small red onion (40g), sliced thinly

20g (¾ ounce) bean sprouts

½ lebanese cucumber (65g), cut into ribbons

⅓ cup fresh coriander leaves (cilantro)

1 Combine garlic, coriander root and stems, ginger, kaffir lime leaves and half the chilli in a mortar and pestle, pound until mixture forms a thick paste. Divide paste in half.

2 Combine half of the paste with prawns and potato in a small bowl; using wet hands form mixture into two patties. Cover, refrigerate 2 hours or overnight.

3 Add half the oil and 2 teaspoons of juice to the remaining paste in a small bowl. Cover, refrigerate until required.

4 Heat remaining oil in a small non-stick frying pan over low heat; cook patties for 3 minutes each side or until cooked through. Transfer to a plate; drizzle patties with remaining juice.

5 Place bread rolls, cut-side down, in same pan for 1 minute or until warm.

6 Toss lettuce, onion, sprouts, cucumber, coriander leaves and remaining chilli through reserved paste. Sandwich salad and patties between rolls.

TIPS Deseed the chillies if you prefer less heat. You can replace prawns with a 200g (6-ounce) firm white fish fillet, such as basa, if you like.

NUTRITIONAL COUNT PER SERVING

● 14.2g total fat   ● 19.1g protein

● 1.8g saturated fat   ● 18.6g fibre

● 1562kJ (373 cal)   ● 403mg sodium

● 34.6g carbohydrate   ● low GI

mixed mushroom trencher with herb salad

PREP + COOK TIME 30 MINUTES ◆ **SERVES** 2

In medieval times a 'trencher' was cut from a round of stale bread and used as a 'plate'.

2 teaspoons rice bran oil

150g (4½ ounces) swiss brown mushrooms, sliced thickly

3 portobello mushrooms (150g), sliced thickly

100g (3 ounces) enoki mushrooms, base trimmed

2 teaspoons fresh lemon thyme leaves

1 small fresh thai red chilli (serrano), seeded, chopped finely

1 clove garlic, crushed

1 teaspoon lemon juice

1 wholemeal sourdough loaf (675g)

1 clove garlic, halved crossways, extra

HERB SALAD

½ teaspoon cumin seeds

1 teaspoon coarsely chopped sunflower seeds

1 teaspoon black chia seeds

2 teaspoons rice bran oil

2 teaspoons lemon juice

½ small red onion (50g), sliced thinly

⅓ cup each fresh flat-leaf parsley and mint leaves

1 tablespoon each fresh dill sprigs and small tarragon leaves

1 Preheat grill (broiler) to high.

2 Make herb salad.

3 Heat oil in a large non-stick frying pan over high heat; cook mushrooms, thyme and chilli, stirring occasionally, for 4 minutes or until browned lightly. Add garlic; cook for 1 minute or until fragrant. Remove from heat, stir through juice. Season with pepper to taste. Cover to keep warm.

4 Cut bread 2cm (¾-inch) from the base lengthways, you will need 175g (5½ ounces) of bread (save the upper portion for another use, see notes). Place bread base on a large oven tray; grill for 1 minute or until toasted lightly. Rub warm bread with extra garlic clove.

5 Top bread with mushrooms and juices; top with salad. Cut in half to serve.

HERB SALAD Heat a large non-stick frying pan over medium heat; cook cumin, sunflower and chia seeds, stirring, for 2 minutes or until seeds are toasted, transfer to a small bowl. Add remaining ingredients; toss to combine.

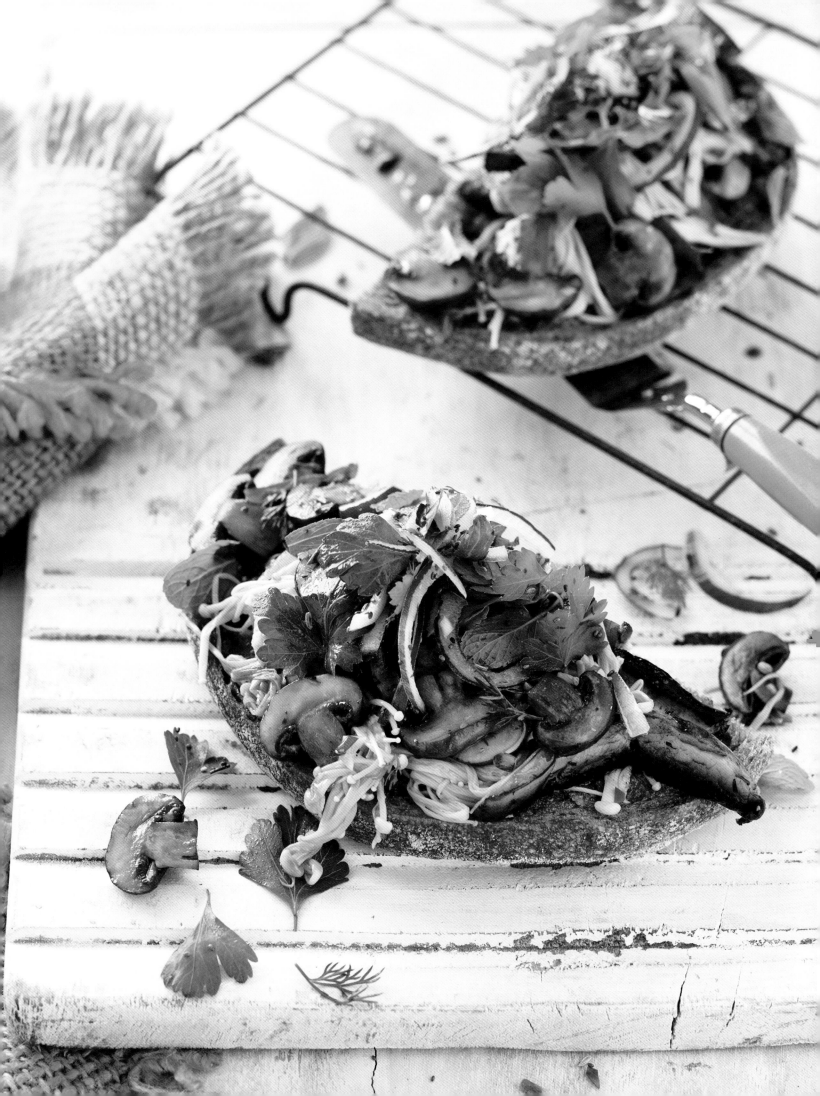

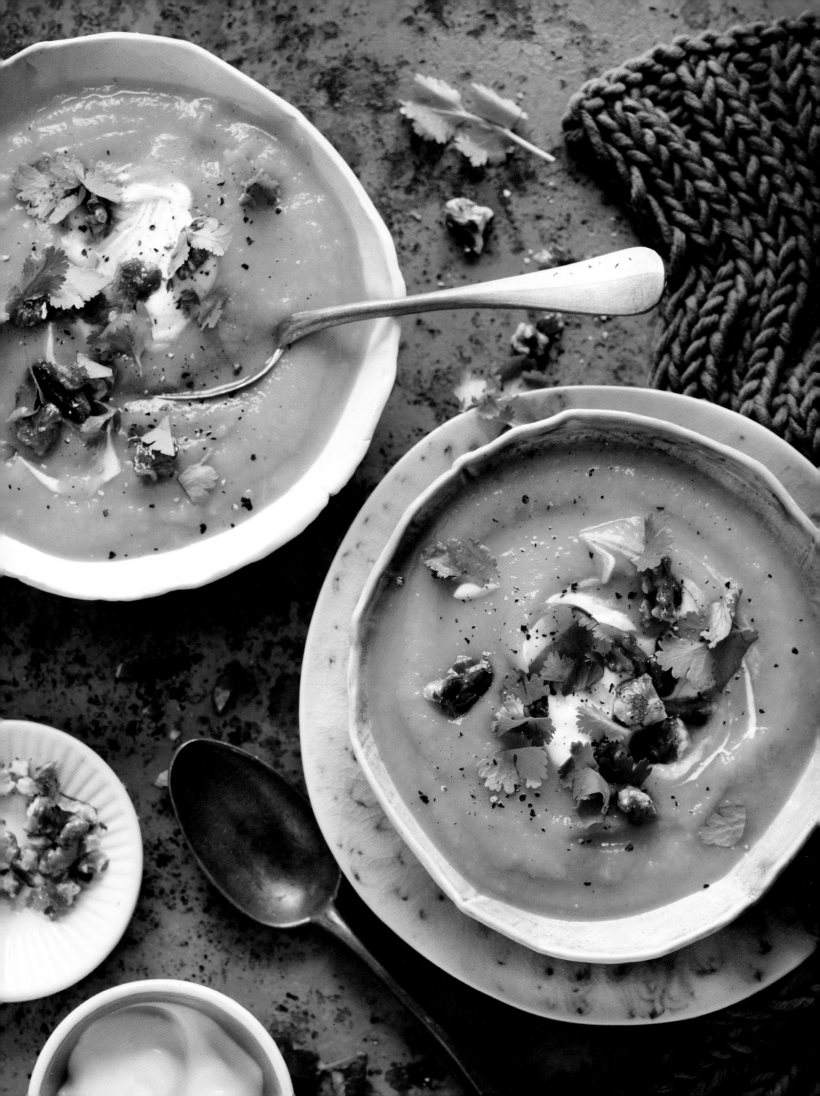

NUTRITIONAL COUNT PER SERVING

- 18.5g total fat
- 3.2g saturated fat
- 1640kJ (392 cal)
- 41.6g carbohydrate
- 10.3g protein
- 11.3g fibre
- 379mg sodium
- medium GI

chai roasted pumpkin soup with honey walnuts

PREP + COOK TIME 50 MINUTES ◆ SERVES 2

1kg (2 pounds) pumpkin, peeled, chopped coarsely

½ teaspoon ground cardamom

¼ teaspoon ground cinnamon

½ teaspoon cracked black pepper

olive-oil spray

¼ cup (25g) walnuts

1 teaspoon honey

2 teaspoons rice bran oil

1 small brown onion (80g), chopped coarsely

2 cloves garlic, sliced

¾ cup (180ml) salt-reduced vegetable stock

1¾ cups (430ml) water

⅓ cup (95g) low-fat greek yoghurt

2 tablespoons roughly chopped fresh coriander leaves (cilantro)

1 Preheat oven to 200°C/400°F. Line a large oven tray with baking paper.

2 Place pumpkin on tray, in a single layer; sprinkle with cardamom, cinnamon and pepper, spray with oil. Roast for 25 minutes or until tender.

3 Meanwhile, line a small oven tray with baking paper. Place nuts on tray, drizzle with honey. Roast for 5 minutes or until golden. Cool.

4 Heat rice bran oil in a large saucepan over medium heat. Cook onion and garlic, stirring, for 5 minutes or until softened. Add pumpkin, stock and the water to the pan; bring to the boil. Remove from heat; cool for 10 minutes.

5 Blend or process pumpkin mixture until smooth. Return pan to heat, stir until hot. To serve, drizzle soup with yoghurt; sprinkle with nuts and coriander.

TIP You can freeze the soup in airtight containers.

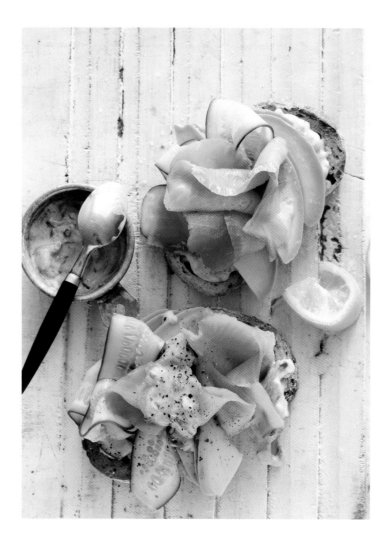
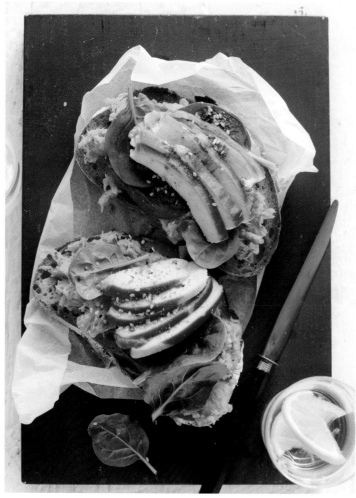

avocado, trout & fennel tzatziki sandwich

PREP TIME 10 MINUTES ◆ **SERVES** 2

Cut a lebanese cucumber in half crossways; cut one half into ribbons using a vegetable peeler. Coarsely grate remaining cucumber and squeeze out excess moisture; combine in a bowl with 2 tablespoons low-fat plain yoghurt and 1 teaspoon ground fennel. Top 2 slices of toasted soy and linseed sourdough evenly with half a small sliced avocado, cucumber ribbons and 60g (2 ounces) smoked trout slices. Drizzle with fennel tzatziki.

TIP Grind fennel seeds in a mortar and pestle or a mini food processor, if ground fennel is unavailable.

NUTRITIONAL COUNT PER SERVING

- 11.9g total fat
- 17.1g protein
- 2.4g saturated fat
- 5.3g fibre
- 1391kJ (332 cal)
- 436mg sodium
- 36.2g carbohydrate
- low GI

chicken and pumpkin open sandwich

PREP + COOK TIME 30 MINUTES ◆ **SERVES** 2

Preheat oven to 220°C/425°F. Line an oven tray with baking paper. Place 200g (6½ ounces) coarsely chopped pumpkin onto tray. Spray with cooking oil and sprinkle with 1 teaspoon dukkah. Bake for 25 minutes or until tender; mash roughly with a fork. Top 2 slices toasted wholemeal sourdough with pumpkin, 20g (¾ ounce) baby spinach leaves and 125g (4 ounces) sliced smoked chicken breast. Drizzle with combined ½ teaspoon macadamia oil and ½ teaspoon dukkah.

NUTRITIONAL COUNT PER SERVING

- 10.1g total fat
- 26.4g protein
- 2g saturated fat
- 7.7g fibre
- 1514kJ (362 cal)
- 405mg sodium
- 37.3g carbohydrate
- low GI

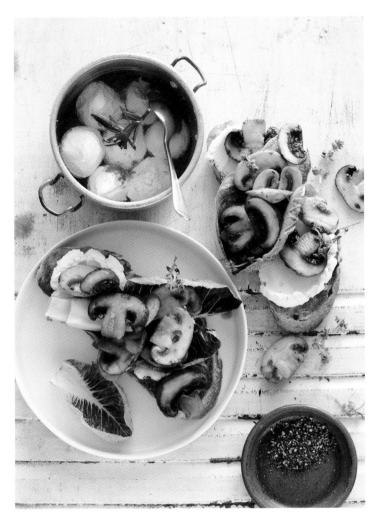

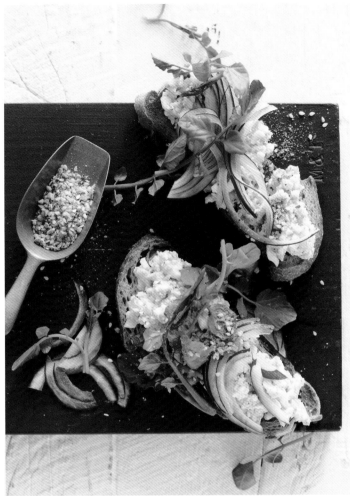

mushroom & labne sandwich

PREP + COOK TIME 15 MINUTES ♦ SERVES 2

Roughly chop 80g (2½ ounces) each swiss brown and button mushrooms. Lightly spray a large non-stick frying pan with cooking oil. Cook mushrooms, 1 crushed garlic clove and 2 teaspoons fresh thyme leaves, over medium heat, for 5 minutes or until browned. Top 2 thin slices of seeded sourdough bread with 2 tablespoons labne, the mushroom mixture, 2 radicchio leaves and an extra 1 tablespoon of labne; drizzle with 2 teaspoons of olive oil.

TIP Labne is a cheese made from strained yoghurt. You can find it at specialty food stores.

middle-eastern egg and cheese sandwich

PREP TIME 10 MINUTES ♦ MAKES 2

Mash 2 hard-boiled eggs with a fork in a medium bowl. Stir in ¼ cup reduced-fat cottage cheese and 1 tablespoon pistachio dukkah. Top 2 slices of toasted rye sourdough with egg mixture, 25g (¾ ounce) watercress sprigs and ¼ thinly sliced small red onion.

TIPS We've used dukkah but you could add curry powder instead for a classic egg sandwich. Pistachio dukkah is available from most major supermarkets in the spice aisle. Store remaining watercress in the fridge with its stems in water, like flowers, for 2 days.

NUTRITIONAL COUNT PER SERVING

- 10.6g total fat
- 11.5g protein
- 2.1g saturated fat
- 6.9g fibre
- 1313kJ (314 cal)
- 413mg sodium
- 39.5g carbohydrate
- low GI

NUTRITIONAL COUNT PER SERVING

- 10.1g total fat
- 19.3g protein
- 2.7g saturated fat
- 5g fibre
- 1418kJ (339 cal)
- 447mg sodium
- 39.7g carbohydrate
- low GI

4 WAYS WITH LENTILS

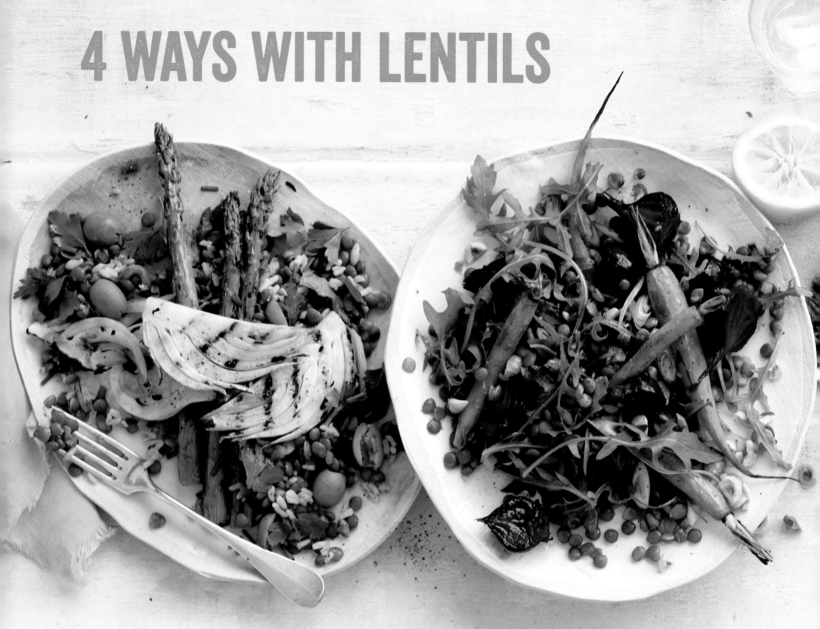

asparagus & fennel salad

PREP + COOK TIME 1 HOUR ◆ **SERVES** 2

Bring ½ cup (100g) dried brown lentils to the boil; simmer, covered, for 45 minutes or until tender, drain. Spray 6 asparagus spears and half a finely sliced fennel bulb with oil; cook on a heated grill plate for 3 minutes or until brown and tender. Combine vegetables in a large bowl with lentils, ½ cup cooked brown rice, ½ cup fresh flat-leaf parsley leaves, ¼ cup toasted pepitas, 2 tablespoons finely chopped fresh chives and ¼ cup sliced green olives. Drizzle with 2 tablespoons lemon juice and 2 teaspoons rice bran oil. Season with pepper.

NUTRITIONAL COUNT PER SERVING

- 21g total fat
- 3.1g saturated fat
- 2023kJ (483 cal)
- 43.8g carbohydrate
- 23.2g protein
- 14.7g fibre
- 267mg sodium
- low GI

beetroot & hazelnut salad

PREP + COOK TIME 1½ HOURS ◆ **SERVES** 2

Bring ⅔ cup (130g) dried brown lentils to the boil; simmer, covered, for 45 minutes or until tender, drain. Preheat oven to 200°C/400°F. Place 1 bunch trimmed and washed baby beetroot (beet) on a large oven tray; cover with foil. Roast for 30 minutes. Add 1 bunch trimmed, peeled baby carrots, spray with olive oil; roast, uncovered, for a further 30 minutes or until tender. Peel and halve beetroot; combine on a serving platter with carrots, lentils, 2 cups baby rocket (arugula), 2 sliced green onions (scallions) and ¼ cup roasted chopped hazelnuts. Drizzle with 2 tablespoons lemon juice and toss gently to combine.

NUTRITIONAL COUNT PER SERVING

- 13.8g total fat
- 0.8g saturated fat
- 1884kJ (450 cal)
- 46.5g carbohydrate
- 22.1g protein
- 24.3g fibre
- 212mg sodium
- low GI

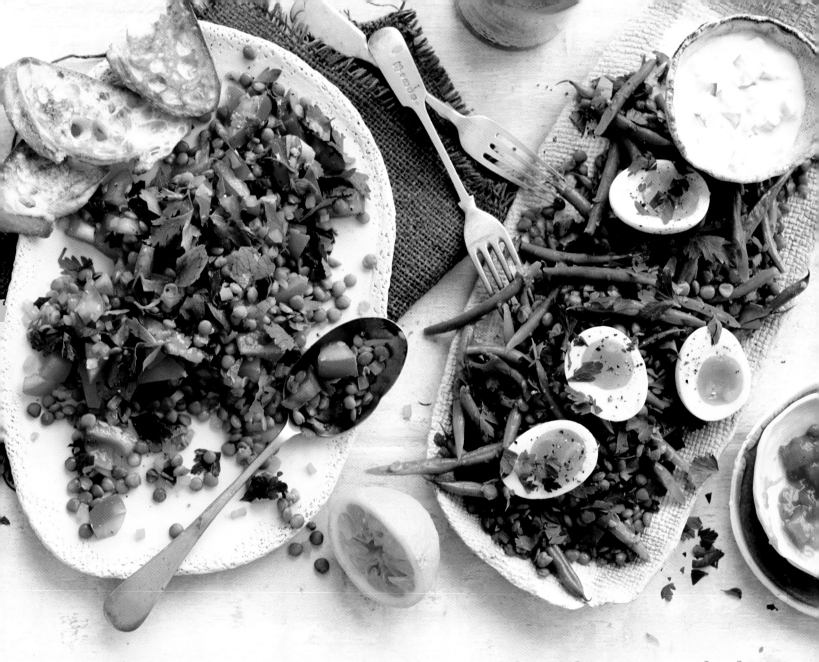

lentil & herb tabbouleh

PREP + COOK TIME 1 HOUR ◆ SERVES 2

Bring ⅓ cup (65g) dried brown lentils to the boil; simmer, covered, for 45 minutes or until tender, drain. Combine 1 finely chopped small yellow capsicum (bell pepper), 2 finely chopped medium tomatoes, ⅔ cup finely chopped fresh flat-leaf parsley, ¼ cup finely chopped fresh mint leaves, 1 teaspoon finely grated lemon rind, 2 tablespoons lemon juice, ¼ teaspoon dried chilli flakes, 1 tablespoon rice bran oil and lentils in a large bowl; toss gently to combine. Accompany each serving with one slice of sourdough bread (25g).

NUTRITIONAL COUNT PER SERVING

- 10.7g total fat
- 1.6g saturated fat
- 1226kJ (293 cal)
- 29.3g carbohydrate
- 14.4g protein
- 10.8g fibre
- 151mg sodium
- low GI

spiced lentil & egg salad

PREP + COOK TIME 1 HOUR ◆ SERVES 2

Bring ⅔ cup (130g) dried brown lentils to the boil; simmer, covered, for 45 minutes or until tender, drain. Cook 2 eggs in boiling water for 6 minutes; cool, shell, then halve eggs. Combine lentils in a bowl with 200g (6½ ounces) blanched sliced green beans and 1 teaspoon curry powder. Top lentil mixture with eggs and 2 tablespoons roughly chopped parsley leaves. Top with ¼ cup light tzatziki and 1 tablespoon mango chutney to serve.

NUTRITIONAL COUNT PER SERVING

- 7.3g total fat
- 1.8g saturated fat
- 1121kJ (289 cal)
- 29.1g carbohydrate
- 22.9g protein
- 10g fibre
- 340mg sodium
- low GI

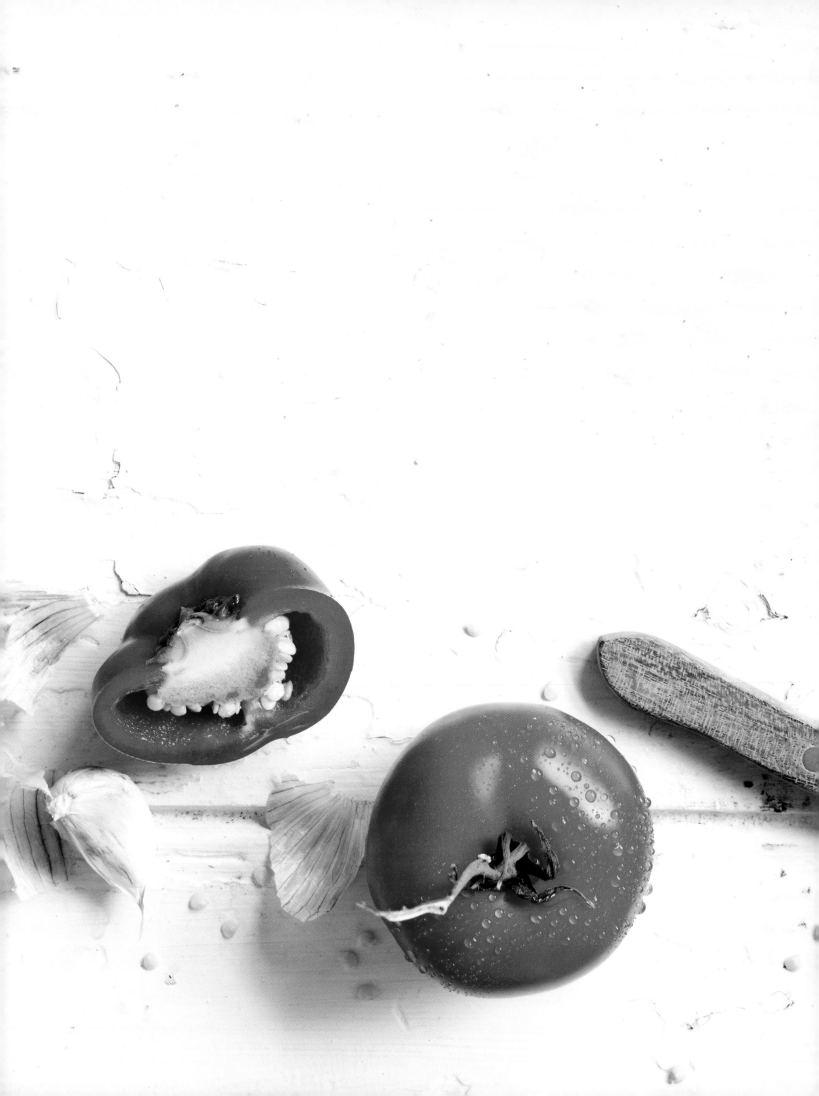

DINNER

Just because you're eating well, it
doesn't mean boring food... these
meals are delicious and healthy.

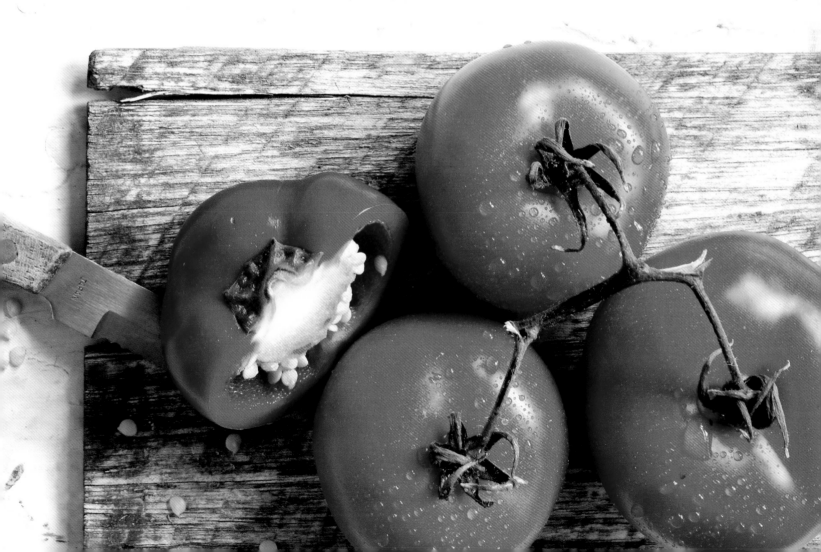

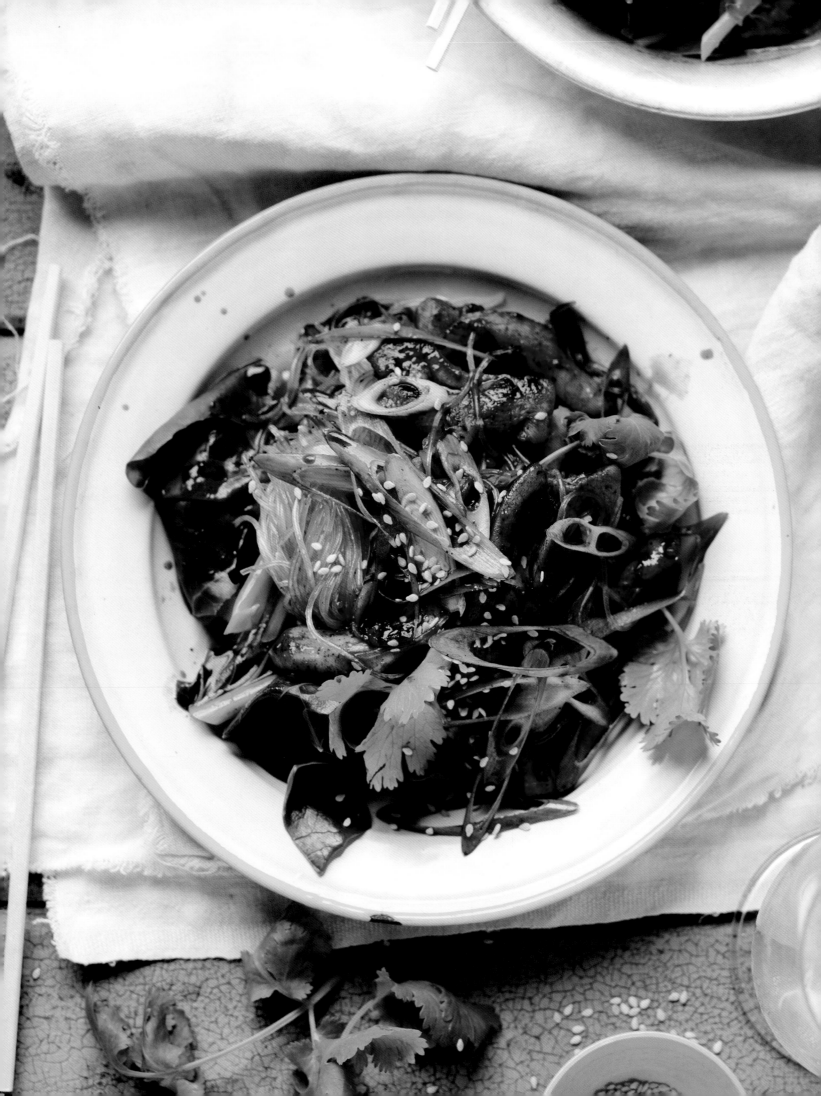

NUTRITIONAL COUNT PER SERVING

● 14.8g total fat ● 28.2g protein
● 3.6g saturated fat ● 5.3g fibre
● 1557kJ (372 cal) ● 449mg sodium;
● 29g carbohydrate ● low GI

sticky chicken with noodles

PREP + COOK TIME 15 MINUTES ◆ SERVES 2

250g (8 ounces) chicken thigh fillets, trimmed, sliced thickly

½ teaspoon chinese five-spice powder

2 teaspoons brown sugar

1 tablespoon sweet chilli sauce

2 teaspoons salt-reduced soy sauce

2 teaspoons olive oil

60g (2 ounces) bean thread vermicelli

300g (9½ ounces) gai lan, trimmed, cut into 5cm (2-inch) lengths

2 tablespoons water

2 green onions (scallions), sliced thinly

2 tablespoons fresh coriander leaves (cilantro)

1 teaspoon sesame seeds, toasted

1 Combine chicken with spice, sugar and half of the sauces in a medium bowl.

2 Heat oil in a wok over high heat; stir-fry chicken mixture, in batches, until chicken is browned and sticky. Remove from wok. Wipe wok clean.

3 Meanwhile, place noodles in a large heatproof bowl, cover with boiling water; stand for 5 minutes or until tender, drain.

4 Add gai lan to wok with the water; stir-fry for 1 minute or until just tender. Add remaining sauces; stir-fry for 1 minute or until heated through. Add noodles to wok; toss until just combined.

5 Top noodles with chicken; sprinkle with onion, coriander and sesame seeds to serve.

TIPS Swap bean thread vermicelli for rice stick noodles. Chicken can be marinated a day ahead; store, covered, in the fridge.

NUTRITIONAL COUNT PER SERVING

- 21.8g total fat
- 6.1g saturated fat
- 2339kJ (559 cal)
- 51.5g carbohydrate
- 35.5g protein
- 6.7g fibre
- 414mg sodium;
- medium GI

stir-fried beef and brown rice with carrot and cucumber pickle

PREP + COOK TIME 20 MINUTES ◆ **SERVES** 2

250g (8-ounce) packet microwave brown rice

1 tablespoon olive oil

2 eggs, beaten lightly

1 clove garlic, crushed

1 tablespoon grated fresh ginger

200g (6½ ounces) lean minced (ground) beef

2 teaspoons oyster sauce

2 cups (160g) shredded cabbage

2 tablespoons shredded fresh mint leaves

1 green onion (scallion), sliced thinly

CARROT AND CUCUMBER PICKLE

⅓ cup (80ml) rice wine vinegar

2 tablespoons caster (superfine) sugar

¼ teaspoon dried chilli flakes

1 small carrot (70g), cut into matchsticks

1 lebanese cucumber (130g), seeded, cut into matchsticks

1 Cook rice according to packet instructions.

2 Meanwhile, make carrot and cucumber pickle.

3 Heat 1 teaspoon of the oil in a wok over high heat; add half the egg, swirl wok to make a thin omelette. Cook, uncovered, until egg is just set. Remove from wok; roll tightly, cut into thick strips. Repeat process with another 1 teaspoon of the oil and remaining egg. Roll tightly; cut into thin strips.

4 Heat remaining oil in wok; stir-fry garlic and ginger until fragrant. Add mince; cook, stirring, until beef is browned. Add sauce; stir-fry until heated through. Remove from wok.

5 Stir-fry cabbage in wok, adding a little water if needed, until tender. Return beef to wok with rice and mint; stir-fry until hot.

6 Drain carrot and cucumber pickle; serve rice topped with pickle, omelette and onion.

CARROT AND CUCUMBER PICKLE Combine vinegar, sugar and chilli flakes in a small bowl; stir until sugar dissolves. Add carrot and cucumber; toss gently to combine.

TIPS Omit the rice and serve the beef and pickle mixtures in lettuce leaves, if you like. To cook your own brown rice you will need to boil 3/4 cup (150g) brown rice in water for 25 minutes or until tender; drain well.

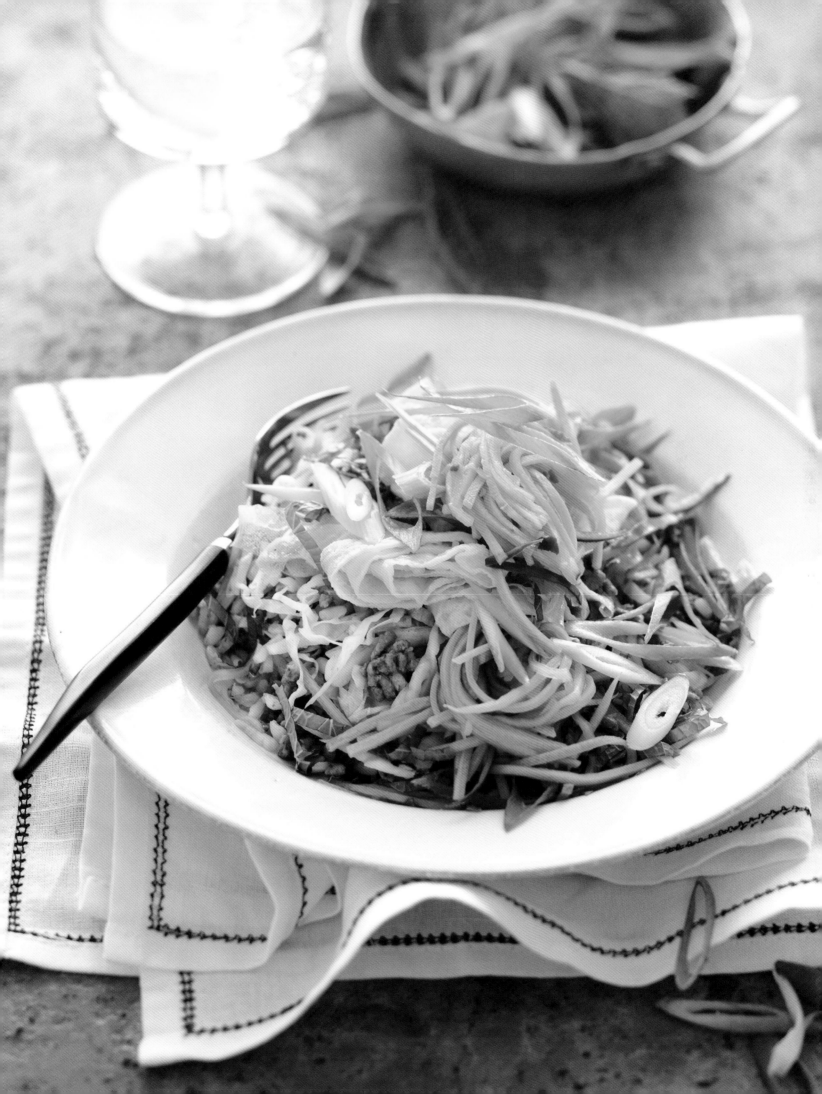

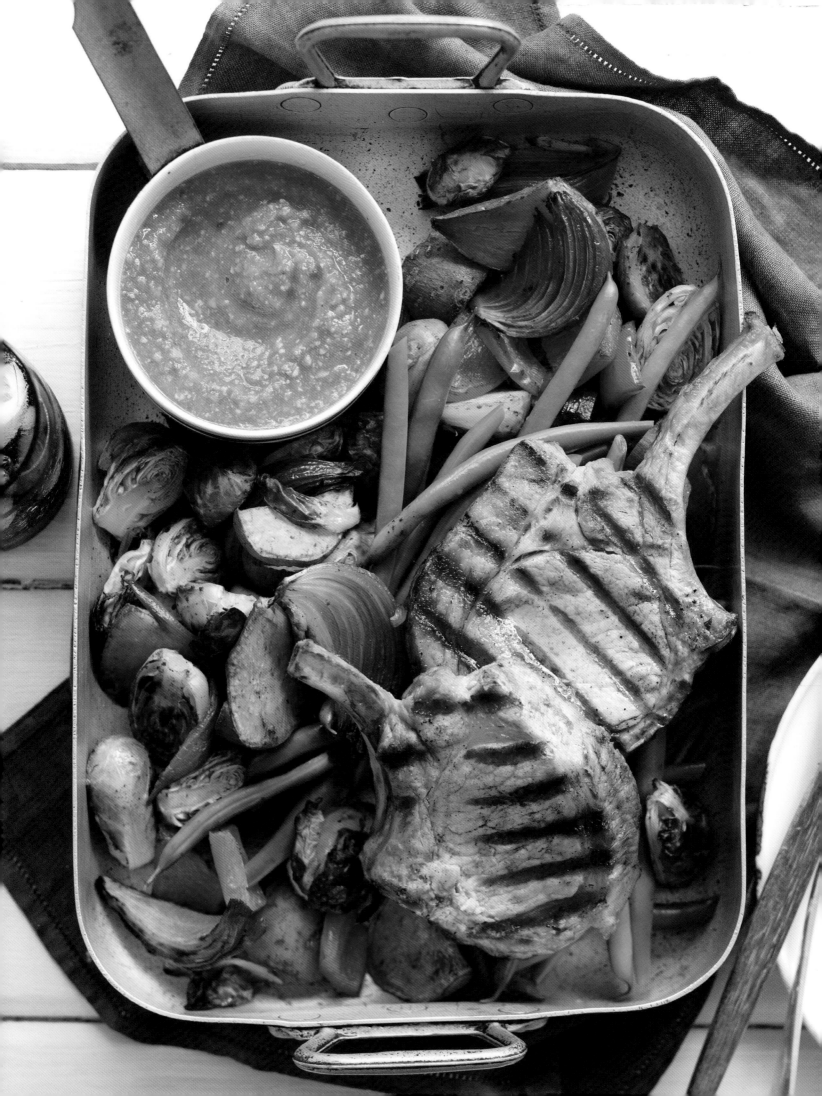

spanish pork cutlets

PREP + COOK TIME 1 HOUR ◆ SERVES 2

1 small kumara (orange sweet potato) (250g), cut into wedges

1 medium red capsicum (bell pepper) (200g), chopped coarsely

200g (6½ ounces) brussels sprouts, halved

1 large red onion (300g), cut into wedges

3 cloves garlic, unpeeled

1 teaspoon smoked paprika

2 teaspoons olive oil

1 medium tomato (150g), quartered

2 pork cutlets (470g), trimmed

200g (6½ ounces) green beans, trimmed

1 tablespoon roasted almond kernels

1 Preheat oven to 220°C/425°F.

2 Combine kumara, capsicum, brussels sprouts, onion and garlic in a large baking dish; sprinkle with paprika and drizzle with half the oil. Toss vegetables to coat. Bake for 40 minutes or until vegetables are golden and tender; add tomato to dish 10 minutes before end of cooking time.

3 Meanwhile, brush pork with remaining oil. Cook pork on a heated grill plate (or grill or barbecue) for 4 minutes each side or until cooked as you like. Remove from heat; cover, rest for 5 minutes.

4 Boil, steam or microwave beans until tender; cover to keep warm.

5 Squeeze garlic from skin. Blend or process garlic, tomato, nuts and half the capsicum until mixture is smooth.

6 Serve pork with roasted vegetables, beans and roasted tomato and almond sauce.

TIPS Make sure the sauce is hot before serving. If not, reheat it for 1 minute in a microwave-safe dish in a microwave on HIGH (100%). This sauce would also go well with roasted chicken. Double this recipe for an easy but impressive dinner for friends.

indian-spiced patties with carrot raita

PREP + COOK TIME 30 MINUTES ◆ **SERVES** 2

420g (13½ ounce) canned no-added salt chickpeas (garbanzo beans), rinsed, drained

1 fresh long green chilli, chopped coarsely

¼ cup firmly packed fresh mint leaves

1½ teaspoons ground cumin

½ teaspoon ground cinnamon

1 clove garlic, crushed

1 teaspoon grated fresh ginger

2 tablespoons water

cooking-oil spray

30g (1 ounce) baby spinach leaves

1 wholemeal pitta bread (80g), warmed

2 lemon wedges

CARROT RAITA

½ cup (140g) low-fat plain yoghurt

½ teaspoon ground cumin

½ small carrot (35g), grated

1 Make carrot raita.

2 Blend or process chickpeas, chilli, mint, cumin, cinnamon, garlic, ginger and the water until just smooth. Shape two level tablespoons of mixture into patties.

3 Lightly spray a large non-stick frying pan with oil; cook patties, over medium heat, for 3 minutes each side or until browned and heated through.

4 Serve patties with the spinach, pitta bread, lemon wedges and raita.

CARROT RAITA Combine ingredients in a small bowl.

TIP If the pattie mixture looks dry when you process it, test it by pinching the mixture with your fingers – it should hold together.

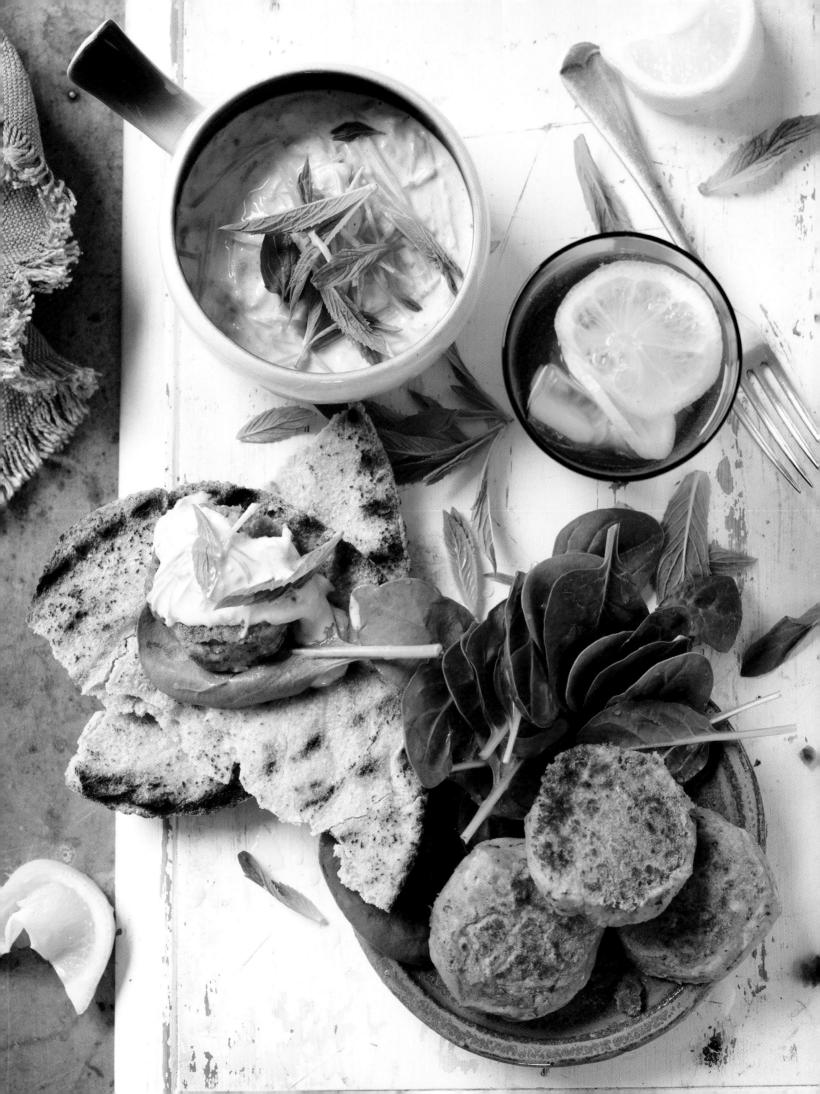

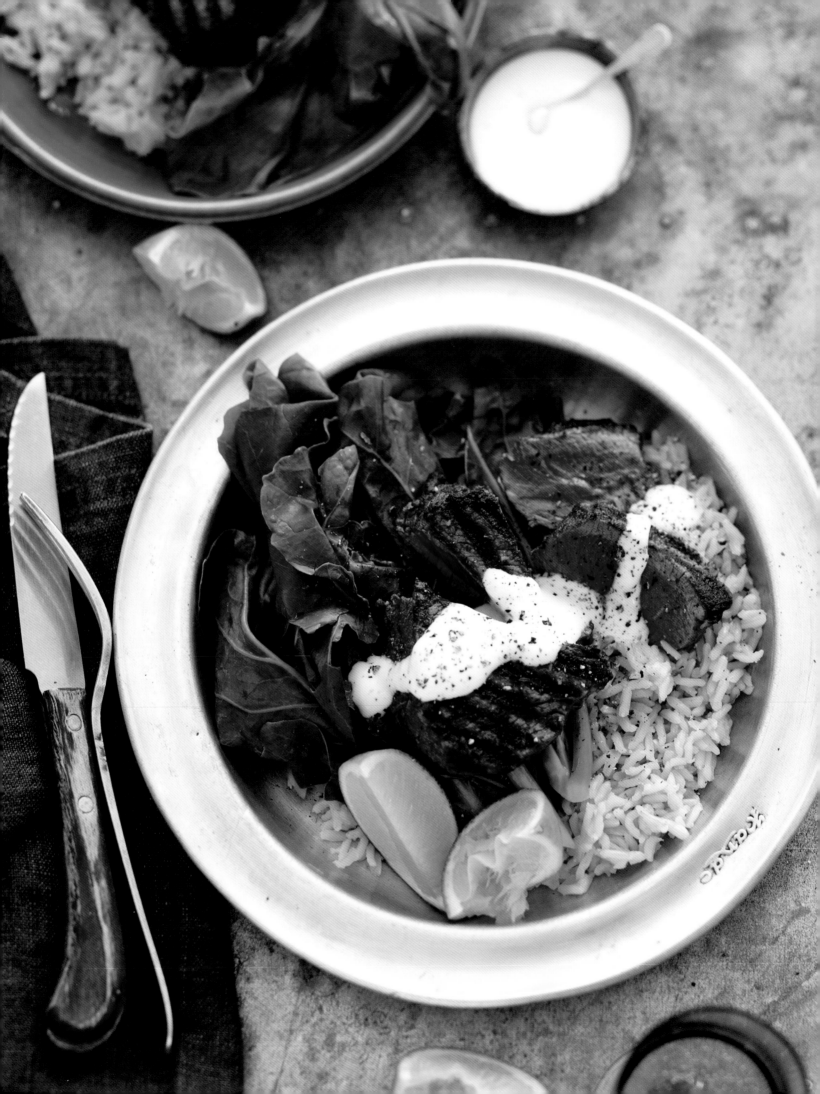

NUTRITIONAL COUNT PER SERVING

● 13.6g total fat ● 39g protein
● 3.8g saturated fat ● 6g fibre
● 1679kJ (401 cal) ● 320mg sodium
● 27.3g carbohydrate ● medium GI

five-spice beef with wasabi sauce

PREP + COOK TIME 20 MINUTES ◆ SERVES 2

2 x 125g (4-ounce) beef eye fillet steaks

1 teaspoon chinese five-spice powder

2 teaspoons olive oil

300g (9½ ounces) gai lan, halved crossways

1 cup (165g) packaged microwave brown basmati rice

2 teaspoons salt-reduced soy sauce

2 lime wedges

WASABI SAUCE

½ cup (140g) low-fat plain yoghurt

½ teaspoon wasabi paste

½ clove garlic, crushed

3 teaspoons lime juice

1 Make the wasabi sauce.

2 Coat steaks in combined five-spice and oil. Cook on a heated grill plate (or grill or barbecue) for 3 minutes each side or until cooked as desired. Cover; rest for 5 minutes.

3 Cook gai lan stems in a saucepan of boiling water for 3 minutes. Add the leaves; cook for 1 minute or until tender, drain.

4 Microwave rice until hot. Serve steaks with rice and gai lan; drizzle soy sauce over gai lan and accompany with lime wedges and wasabi sauce.

WASABI SAUCE Combine ingredients in a small bowl.

TIPS You can add more or less wasabi to the sauce depending on your heat preference – watch the sodium level if adding extra. Raw brown basmati rice can be difficult to find, though both major supermarkets stock the microwave brands. If cooking your own rice, you will need 1/2 cup uncooked brown basmati rice.

jerk salmon with black bean salad

PREP + COOK TIME 25 MINUTES ◆ SERVES 2

1 teaspoon ground coriander

½ teaspoon dried thyme

¼ teaspoon each ground cinnamon, chilli powder and allspice

1 clove garlic, crushed

2 x 100g (3-ounce) salmon fillets, skin and bones removed

1 trimmed cob corn (250g)

cooking-oil spray

½ cup (100g) canned black beans, rinsed, drained

100g (3 ounces) cherry tomatoes, halved

½ small avocado (100g), chopped coarsely

1 green onion (scallion), sliced thinly

½ cup loosely packed fresh coriander leaves (cilantro)

2 teaspoons olive oil

2 teaspoons lime juice

1 Combine ground coriander, dried thyme, cinnamon, chilli, allspice and garlic in a small bowl; rub all over salmon.

2 Meanwhile, cook corn in boiling water for 6 minutes or until tender. Drain; cool.

3 Lightly spray a large non-stick frying pan with oil. Cook salmon, over medium heat, for 3 minutes each side or until just cooked.

4 Meanwhile, remove kernels from corn. Combine corn with beans, tomato, avocado, onion, coriander and combined olive oil and lime juice in a large bowl.

5 Serve salmon with salad; accompany with lime wedges, if you like.

TIPS Add more chilli powder to the spice mix if you like it hot. Black beans are available from specialty food stores. You can substitute kidney or cannellini beans, if you like – just be aware the sodium level of canned beans can be high, try to buy low-sodium wherever possible.

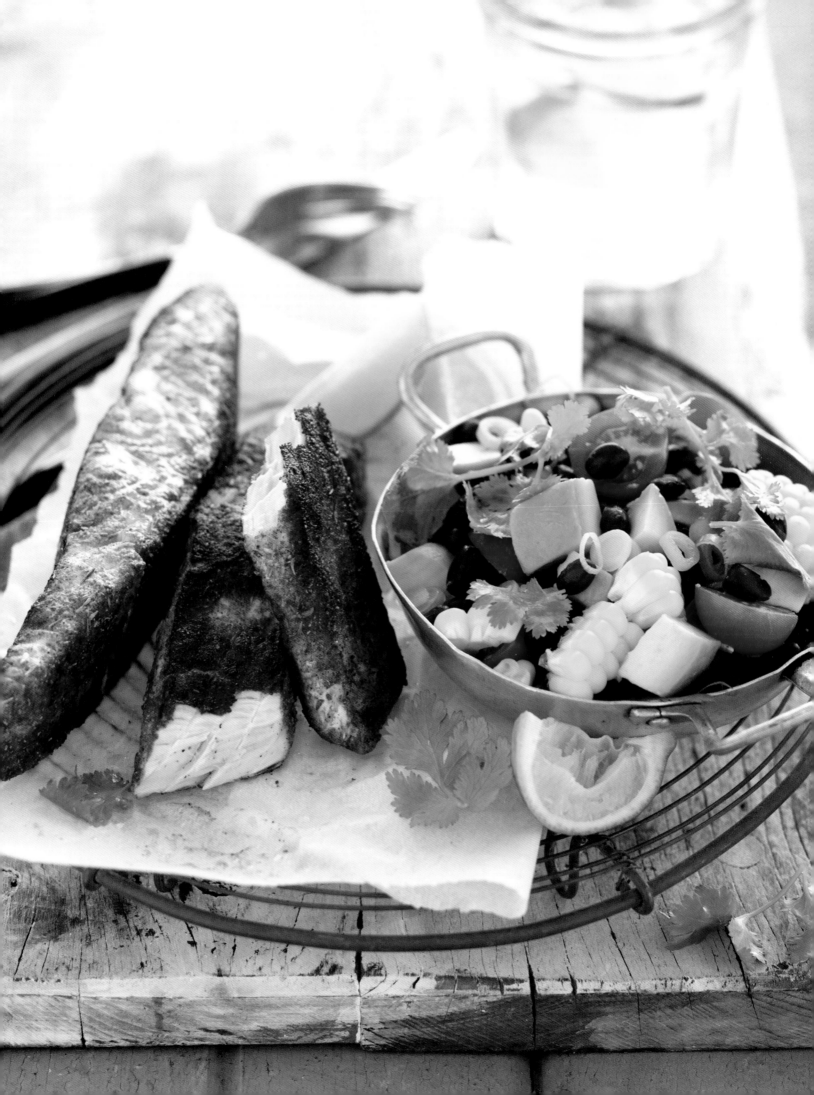

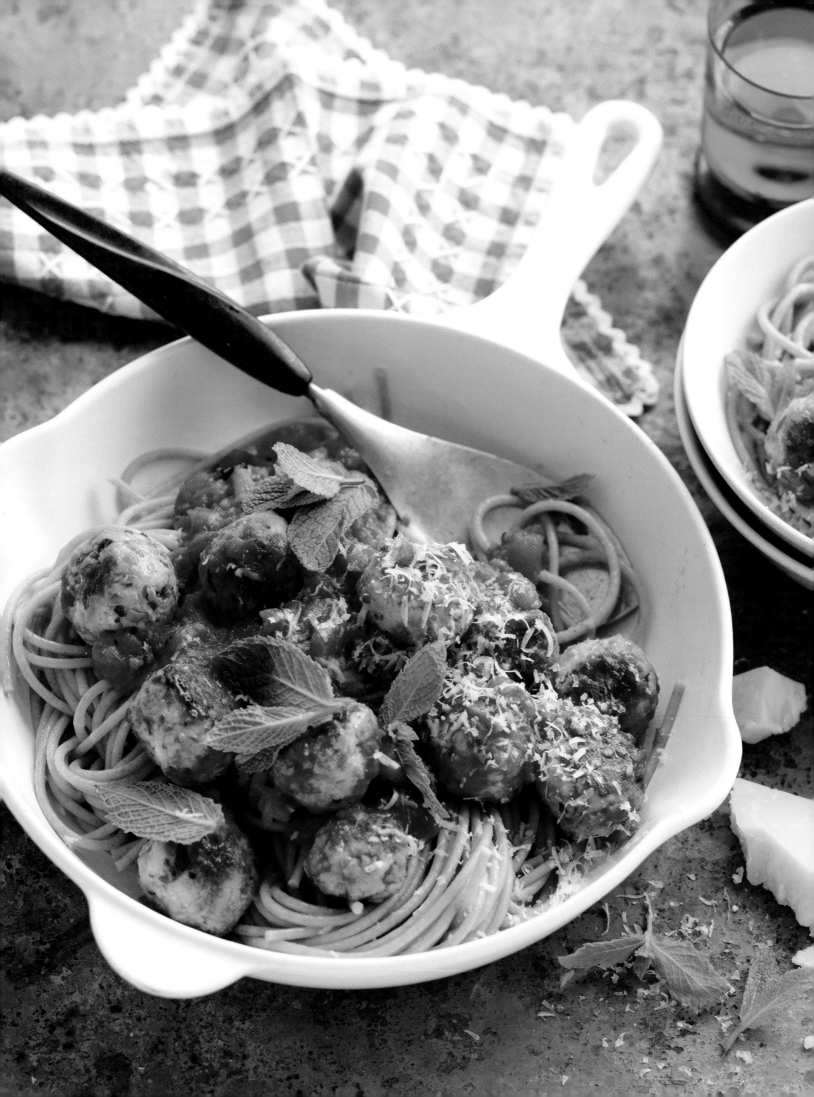

chicken, minted pea and ricotta meatballs

PREP + COOK TIME 50 MINUTES ◆ **SERVES** 2

⅓ **cup (40g) frozen peas**

1 teaspoon finely grated lemon rind

2 tablespoons roughly chopped fresh mint leaves

175g (5½ ounces) minced (ground) chicken

1 clove garlic, crushed

¼ **cup (25g) dried multigrain breadcrumbs**

1 egg yolk

2 tablespoons low-fat ricotta

1 tablespoon olive oil

400g (12½ ounces) canned diced tomatoes

2 teaspoons balsamic vinegar

130g (4 ounces) wholemeal spaghetti

2 tablespoons fresh mint leaves, extra

2 tablespoons shaved parmesan

1 Preheat oven to 240°C/475°F. Grease and line a small shallow baking dish with baking paper.

2 Place the peas in a medium heatproof bowl, cover with boiling water; stand for 1 minute, drain, reserving 1 tablespoon of the water. Blend or process peas, reserved water, rind and chopped mint until just combined.

3 Combine chicken, garlic, breadcrumbs and egg yolk in a medium bowl, mix well. Stir in pea mixture and ricotta.

4 Roll level tablespoons of mixture into balls using wet hands. Place in prepared dish; drizzle with oil. Roast for 15 minutes, turning once. Add tomato and vinegar; cook for 5 minutes or until the meatballs are cooked through and sauce is hot.

5 Meanwhile, cook pasta in a large saucepan of boiling water until just tender. Drain.

6 Serve pasta with meatballs and sauce. Top with extra mint and cheese.

TIP You can make the meatballs ahead of time and freeze them raw or cooked. Defrost the meatballs in the fridge before cooking.

salmon parcels with kipfler potatoes

PREP + COOK TIME 50 MINUTES ◆ SERVES 2

300g (9½ ounces) kipfler potatoes (fingerlings), sliced thinly

1 small red onion, cut into wedges

2 teaspoons olive oil

½ lemon (70g), sliced thinly

1 small tomato (90g), sliced thinly

2 x 150g (9½-ounce) salmon fillets, skin and bones removed

2 teaspoons baby capers, rinsed, drained

1 teaspoon fennel seeds

100g (3 ounces) baby spinach leaves

¼ cup firmly packed fresh parsley leaves

1 Preheat oven to 200°C/400°F.

2 Combine potatoes and onion in a medium baking dish; drizzle with half the oil. Roast for 30 minutes or until browned lightly and tender.

3 Meanwhile, arrange lemon and tomato on two 30cm-square (12-inch square) pieces of baking paper; top with salmon, capers and seeds, drizzle with remaining oil. Fold paper into a parcel to enclose salmon; place on a baking tray. Bake for 8 minutes or until salmon is cooked as you like.

4 Toss spinach through potato mixture.

5 Serve fish with potatoes and spinach and top with parsley.

TIPS Baking the salmon in a parcel means all the flavours, juices and steam are locked in to give a moist and tasty end result. You could try this recipe with firm white fish fillets or even chicken breast. The cooking time will vary depending on the thickness of the cut. You could also try the low-GI Carisma potatoes for this recipe.

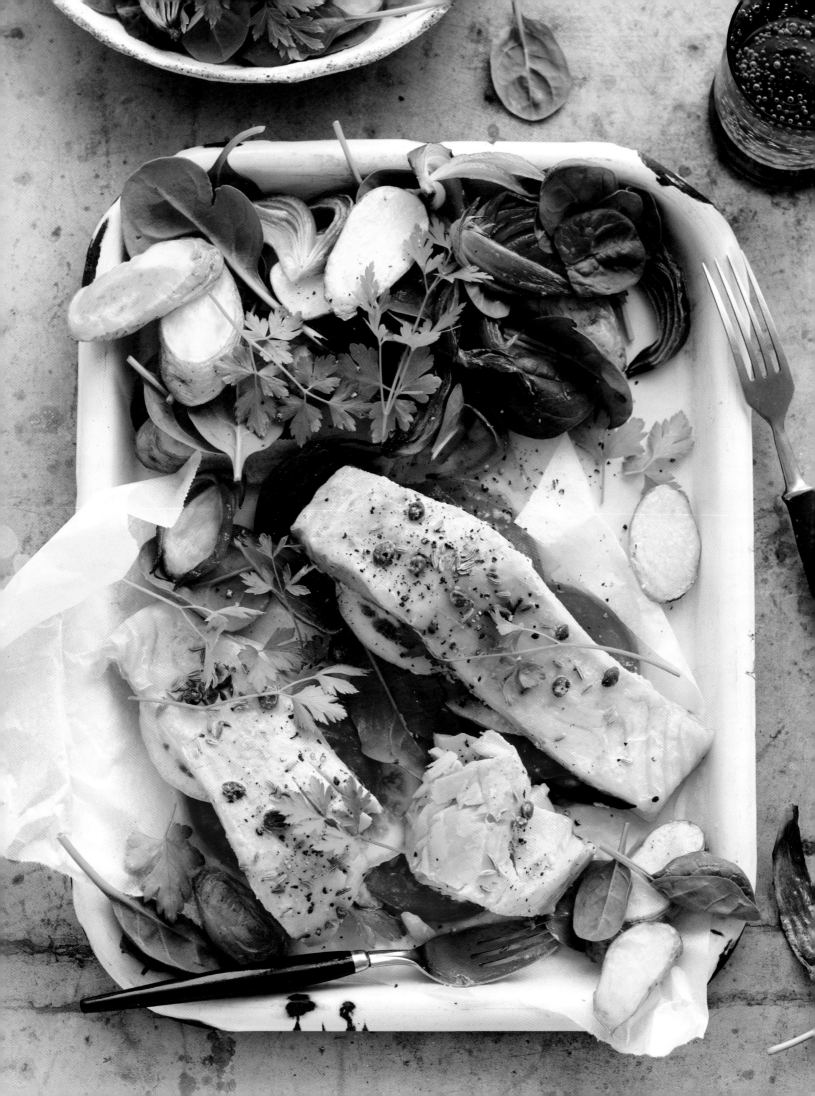

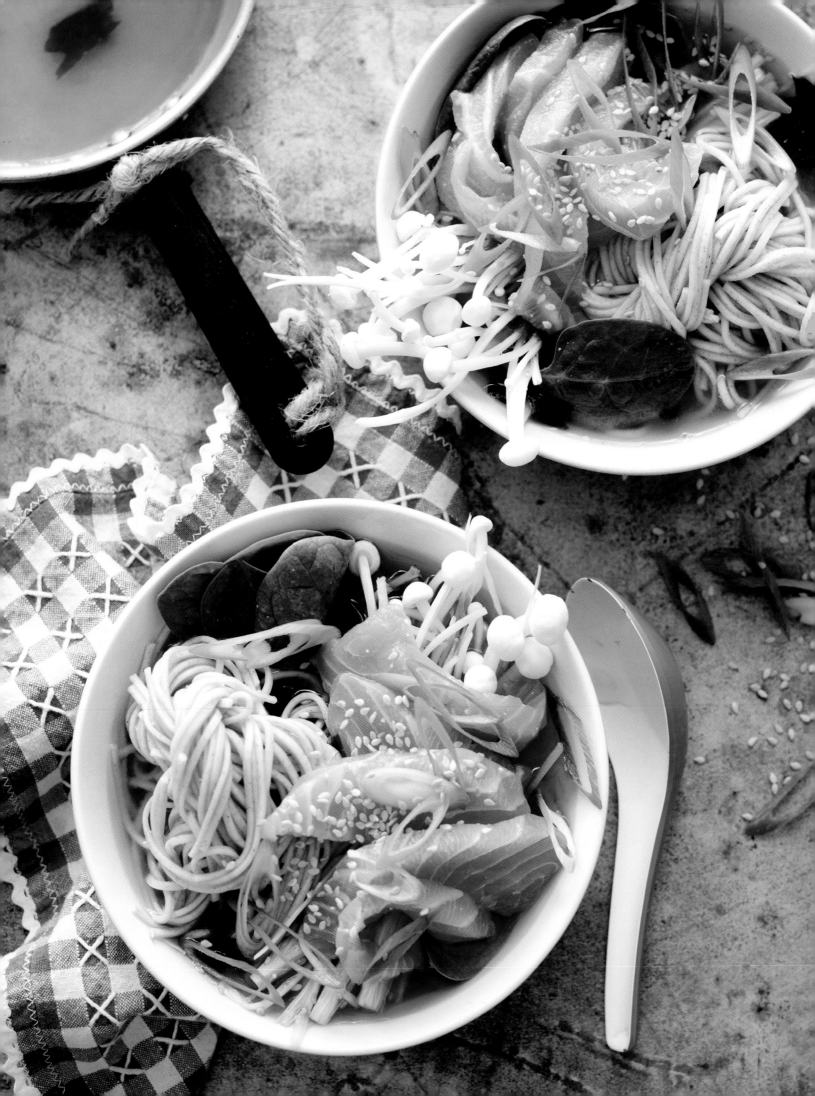

miso broth with salmon and soba

PREP + COOK TIME 25 MINUTES ◆ SERVES 2

70g (2½ ounces) soba noodles

1 teaspoon sesame oil

¾ teaspoon white miso paste

2 cups (500ml) water

50g (1½ ounces) snow peas, sliced thinly

100g (3 ounces) baby spinach leaves

100g (3 ounces) enoki mushrooms, trimmed

120g (4 ounces) sashimi grade salmon, sliced thinly across the grain

1 teaspoon sesame seeds, toasted

1 green onion (scallion), sliced thinly

1   Cook noodles in simmering water for 3 minutes; drain. Rinse under cold water; drain. Toss noodles with oil in a small bowl.

2   Combine miso and the water in a small saucepan; stir over high heat until mixture just comes to the boil. Remove from heat.

3   Divide noodles, snow peas, spinach, mushrooms and salmon evenly between two serving bowls; pour over the hot broth. Sprinkle with seeds and shallots; serve immediately.

TIPS You can sear the salmon on all sides and finely slice it before adding it to the soup. The salmon can be substituted with tuna or ocean trout.

NUTRITIONAL COUNT PER SERVING

● 13.7g total fat   ● 40.5g protein

● 3.2g saturated fat   ● 10.3g fibre

● 2095kJ (500 cal)   ● 184mg sodium;

● 47g carbohydrate   ● low GI

turkish chicken kebabs

PREP + COOK TIME 30 MINUTES (+ REFRIGERATION) ◆ **SERVES** 2

1 cup (280g) low-fat plain yoghurt

1 clove garlic, crushed

1 teaspoon ground cumin

300g (9½ ounces) chicken thigh fillets, trimmed, cut into 3cm (1¼-inch) cubes

2 tablespoons fresh flat-leaf parsley leaves

TOMATO WHEAT PILAF

2 teaspoons olive oil

1 small brown onion (80g), chopped finely

¾ cup (120g) cracked wheat

1½ cups (325ml) water

1 tablespoon salt-reduced tomato paste

CUCUMBER SALAD

½ lebanese cucumber (65g), sliced thinly

1 medium tomato (150g), sliced thinly

¼ small red onion (25g), sliced thinly

1 Combine yoghurt and garlic in a shallow bowl; reserve half the mixture. Stir cumin into remaining yoghurt mixture; add chicken, rub all over to coat in mixture. Cover, refrigerate for 30 minutes.

2 Meanwhile, make tomato wheat pilaf and cucumber salad.

3 Thread chicken equally onto 4 small skewers. Cook chicken on a heated oiled grill plate (or grill or barbecue) for 8 minutes, turning occasionally, or until cooked through.

4 Serve chicken skewers with cucumber salad, reserved garlic yoghurt, tomato wheat pilaf and parsley leaves.

TOMATO WHEAT PILAF Heat oil in a medium saucepan over medium-high heat; cook onion, stirring, for 3 minutes or until softened. Stir in wheat, the water and paste. Bring to the boil, then reduce heat; simmer, covered, for 15 minutes or until liquid is absorbed. Remove from heat; stand, covered, for 10 minutes.

CUCUMBER SALAD Combine ingredients in a small bowl.

TIPS This easy cracked wheat pilaf is a great side for any barbecued meat or fish. If reheating leftover pilaf, add a little boiling water as it tends to thicken when standing. You can marinate the chicken a day ahead; store, covered, in the fridge. You could add some ground coriander and a pinch of ground chilli to the marinade.

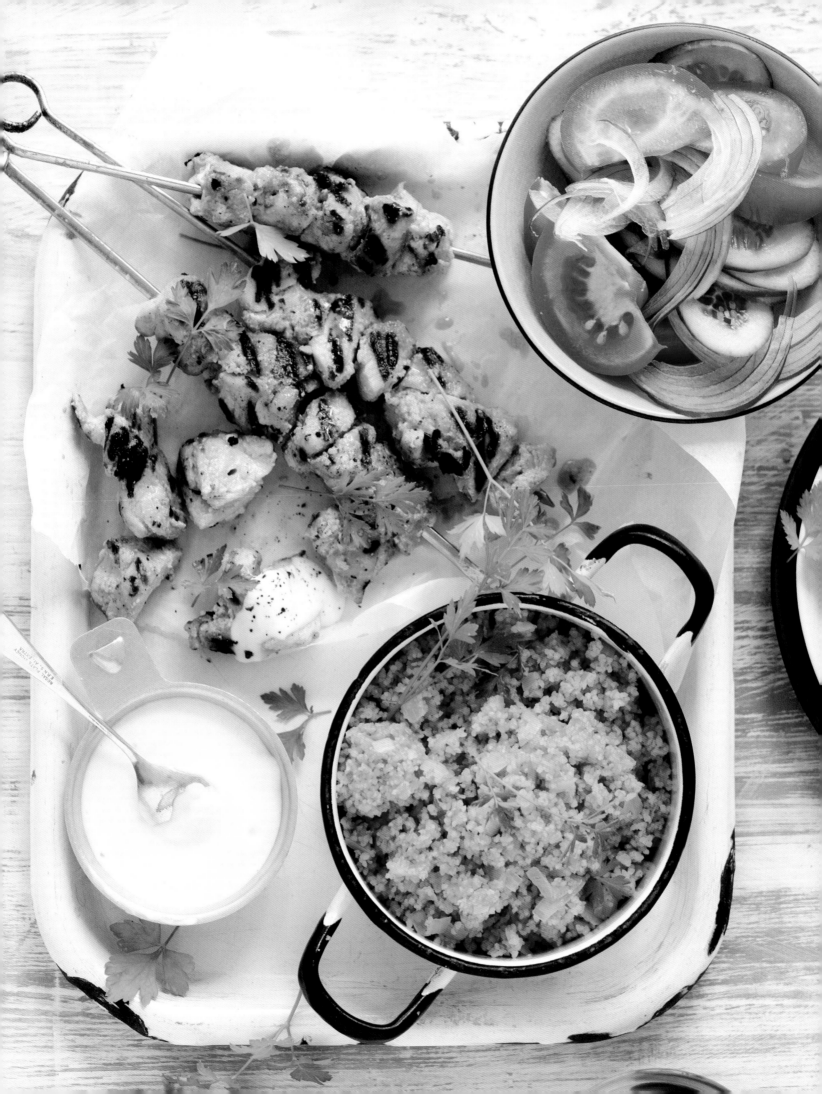

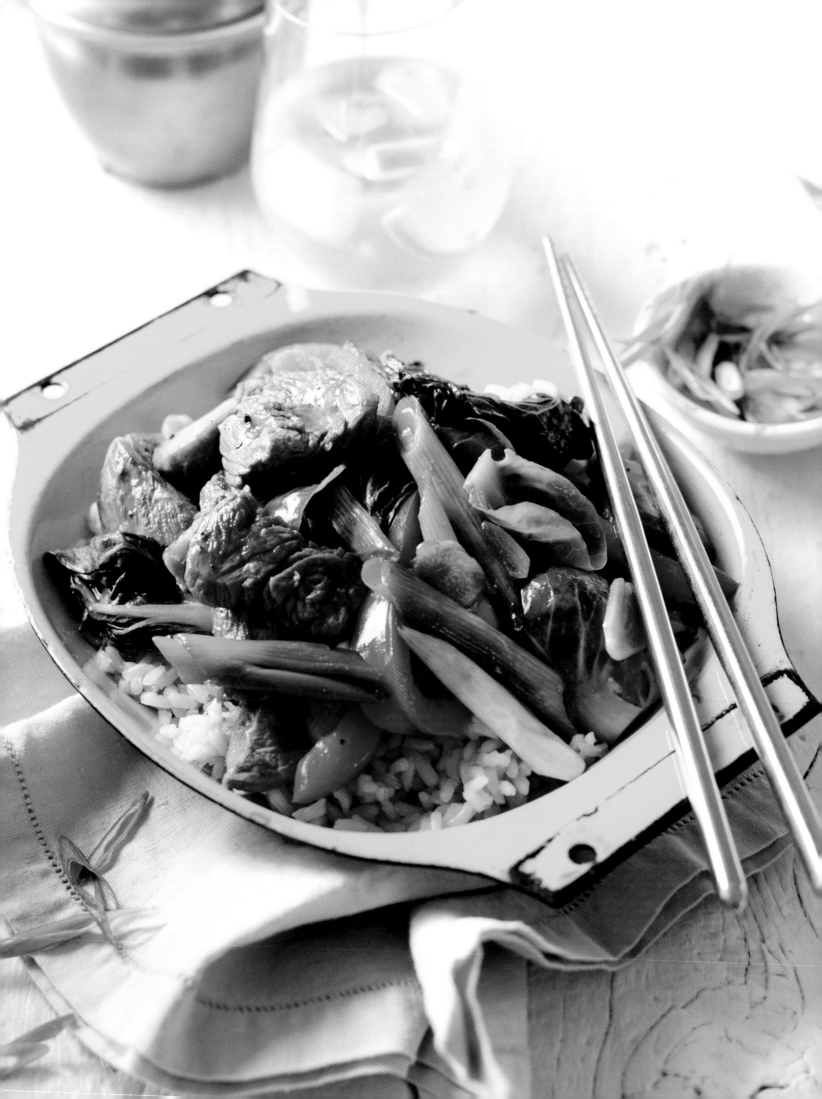

pepper beef stir-fry with brussels sprouts

PREP + COOK TIME 30 MINUTES ◆ SERVES 2

1 tablespoon peanut oil

200g (6½ ounces) brussels sprouts, halved

⅓ cup (80ml) water

1 medium red capsicum (bell pepper) (200g), sliced thinly

3 green onions (scallions), sliced thickly

4 cloves garlic, sliced thinly

250g (7 ounces) beef rump steak, trimmed, cut into 1cm (½-inch) slices

100g (3 ounces) roughly chopped buk choy leaves

1½ tablespoons hoisin sauce

1 tablespoon water, extra

½ teaspoon freshly ground black pepper

250g (8-ounce) packet microwave brown rice

1 Heat 1 teaspoon of the oil in a wok over high heat; stir-fry brussels sprouts for 4 minutes or until browned lightly. Add the water; cook, covered, over medium heat, for 5 minutes or until bright green and just tender. Remove from pan; cover to keep warm.

2 Wipe wok clean. Heat 1 teaspoon of the oil over high heat; stir-fry capsicum and onion for 3 minutes or until browned lightly. Add garlic; stir-fry 1 minute. Add mixture to brussels sprouts; cover to keep warm.

3 Wipe wok clean. Heat remaining oil over high heat; stir-fry beef, in two batches, for 1 minute or until browned. Return vegetables to wok with buk choy, sauce, extra water and pepper; stir-fry 1 minute or until hot.

4 Serve stir-fry with brown rice.

TIPS To cook your own brown rice you will need to boil 3/4 cup (150g) brown rice in water for about 25 minutes or until tender; drain well. Don't cut the beef into thin strips or it will overcook and become tough. You could make this stir-fry with lamb instead of beef.

NUTRITIONAL COUNT PER SERVING

- 22.2g total fat
- 4.5g saturated fat
- 1767kJ (422 cal)
- 33.1g carbohydrate

- 17.5g protein
- 15g fibre
- 309mg sodium
- low GI

ribollita

PREP + COOK TIME 1 HOUR (+ STANDING) ◆ SERVES 2

100g (3 ounces) dried cannellini beans

2 tablespoons extra-virgin olive oil

1 medium carrot (120g), cut into 1cm (½-inch) pieces

1 small red onion (100g), cut into 1cm (½-inch) pieces

1 trimmed celery stalk (100g), cut into 1cm (½-inch) pieces

1 clove garlic, sliced finely

4 large roma (egg) tomatoes (360g), seeded, cut into 1cm (½-inch) pieces

2 medium silver beet leaves (swiss chard) (130g), white stem discarded, chopped coarsely

3½ cups (875ml) water

50g (1½ ounce) rye sourdough, crust removed, torn into bite-size pieces

2 tablespoons finely grated parmesan

1 Place beans in a medium bowl, cover with water; stand overnight. Drain; rinse under cold water, drain. Cook beans in a medium saucepan of boiling water for 40 minutes or until tender. Drain.

2 Meanwhile, heat half the oil in a medium saucepan over low heat; add carrot, onion, celery and garlic. Cook, stirring occasionally, for 20 minutes or until vegetables are softened. Stir in tomato.

3 Increase heat to medium; simmer for 10 minutes.

4 Mash half the cannellini beans with a fork; add to saucepan with remaining beans, silver beet and the water. Simmer for 20 minutes. Remove from heat; fold through bread.

5 Serve soup with parmesan; drizzle with the remaining oil.

TIPS Fold the bread through the hot soup just before serving – this style of soup is very thick. The soup, without the bread, can be made a day ahead; store, covered, in the fridge. You can replace the dried beans with rinsed and drained canned beans; just be aware that canned beans are high in sodium.

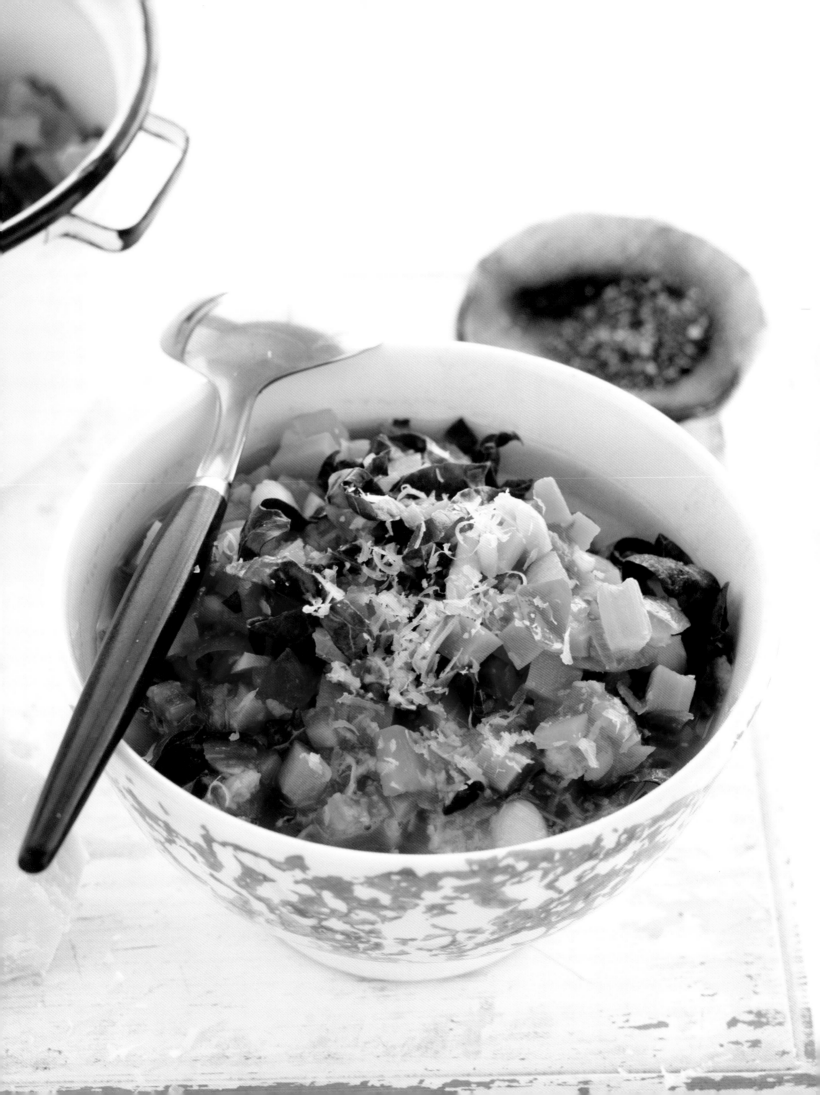

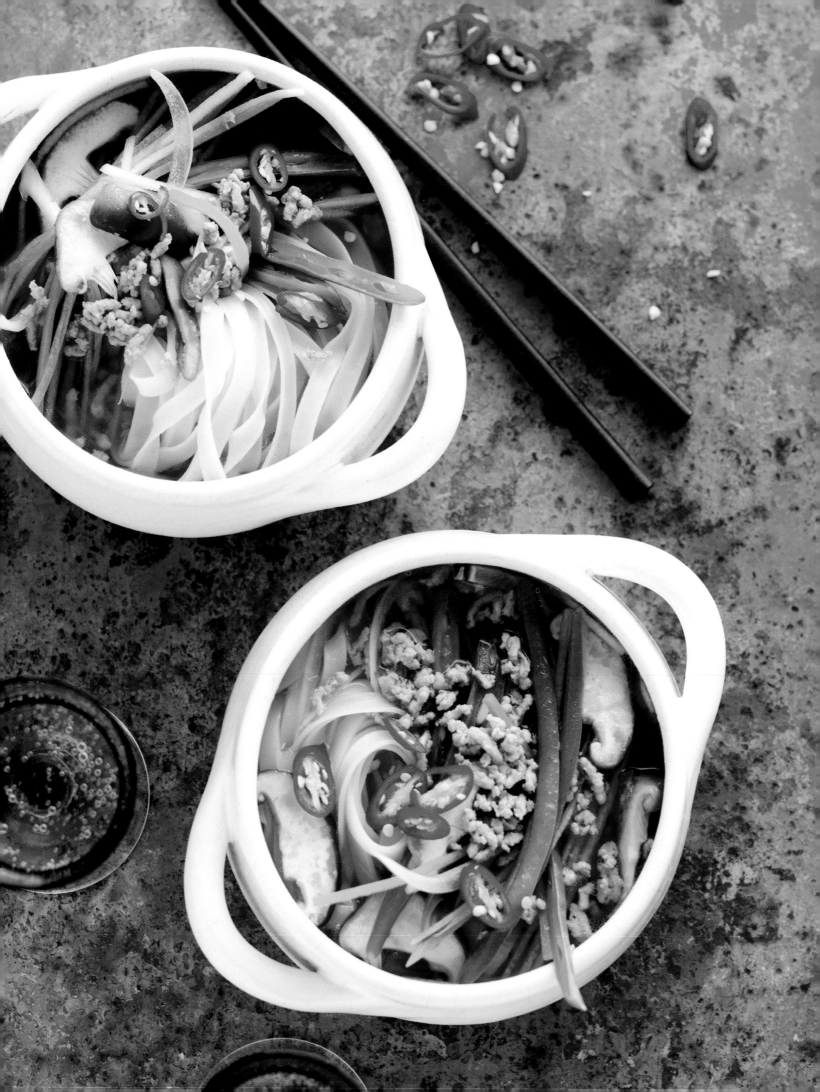

NUTRITIONAL COUNT PER SERVING

● 14.8g total fat
● 3.6g saturated fat
● 1557kJ (372 cal)
● 29g carbohydrate

● 28.2g protein
● 5.3g fibre
● 449mg sodium;
● low GI

japanese-style pork and vegetable soup

PREP + COOK TIME 15 MINUTES ◆ SERVES 2

2 teaspoons canola oil

120g (4 ounces) lean minced (ground) pork

3 teaspoons instant dashi

1 small carrot (70g), cut into matchsticks

½ small brown onion (40g), sliced thinly

60g (1½ ounces) green beans, trimmed, cut into 3cm (1¼-inch) lengths

1 litre (4 cups) water

50g (1½ ounces) small daikon, cut into matchsticks

40g (1½ ounce) fresh shiitake mushrooms, stems removed, sliced thinly

1 fresh small red thai chilli (serrano), sliced thinly

60g (2 ounces) dried rice stick noodles

1 teaspoon sesame oil

1 Heat oil in a medium saucepan over medium heat; cook pork, stirring, for 5 minutes or until cooked.

2 Add dashi, carrot, onion, beans and the water; increase heat to high. Bring to the boil, then reduce heat; simmer for 3 minutes. Add daikon, mushroom and chilli, stir to combine; remove from heat.

3 Meanwhile, cook noodles in a medium saucepan of boiling water according to packet directions; drain.

4 Divide noodles between bowls; top with soup, then drizzle with sesame oil.

TIP Swap pork for chicken if you like.

grilled steak with salsa verde and soft polenta

PREP + COOK TIME 40 MINUTES ◆ SERVES 2

2⅓ cups (580ml) water

½ cup (85g) polenta

1 tablespoon finely grated parmesan

2 x 120g (4-ounce) lean beef eye-fillet steaks

SALSA VERDE

¼ cup firmly packed fresh flat-leaf parsley leaves

2 tablespoons fresh mint leaves

¼ cup firmly packed fresh basil leaves

2 teaspoons rinsed, drained capers

1 clove garlic, crushed

2 teaspoons finely grated lemon rind

1½ tablespoons olive oil

1 Make salsa verde.

2 Boil the water in a medium saucepan. Gradually add polenta, stirring constantly. Reduce heat; simmer, stirring, for 10 minutes or until polenta thickens. Add cheese, stir until cheese melts. Fold through half the salsa verde; cover to keep warm.

3 Meanwhile, cook beef on a heated oiled grill plate (or grill or barbecue) for 4 minutes each side or until browned and cooked as desired. Cover; rest for 5 minutes then slice beef thickly on an angle.

4 Serve beef with polenta; accompany with remaining salsa verde.

SALSA VERDE Blend or process parsley, mint, basil, capers, garlic and rind until a coarse paste forms. Transfer to a small bowl; stir in oil to combine.

TIP The polenta will firm on standing, so stir in a little hot water to loosen the mixture.

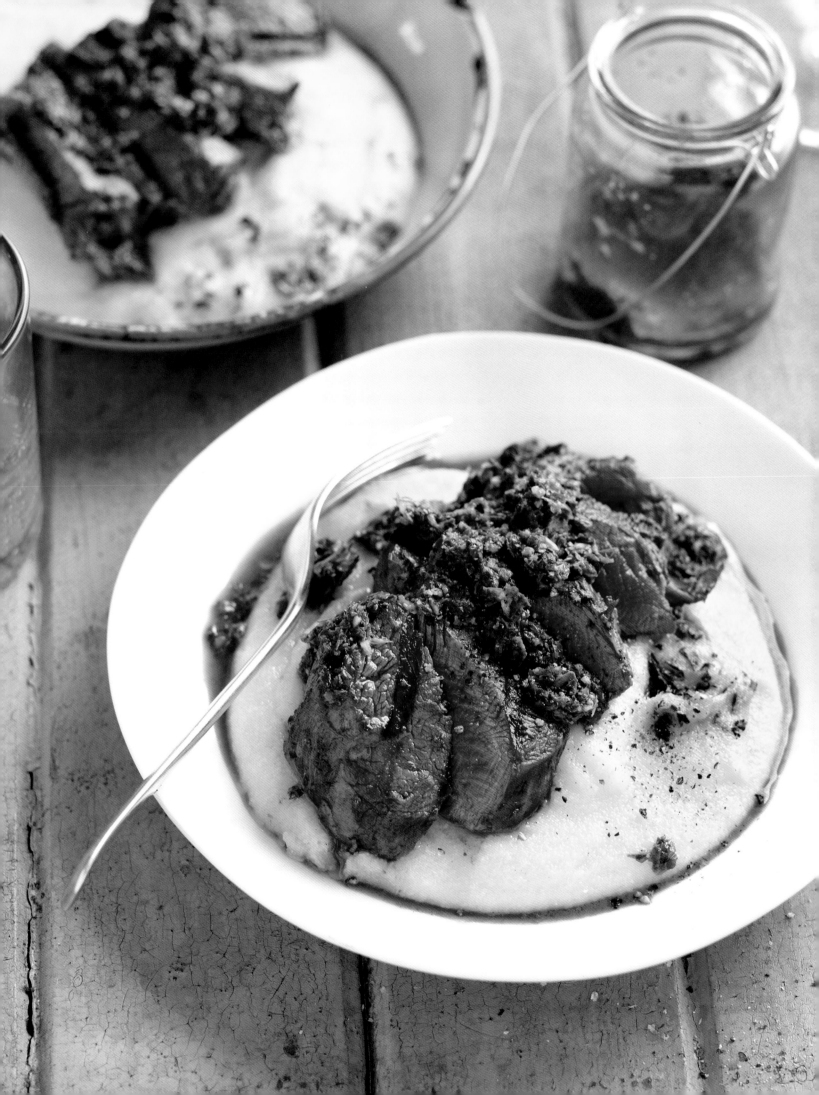

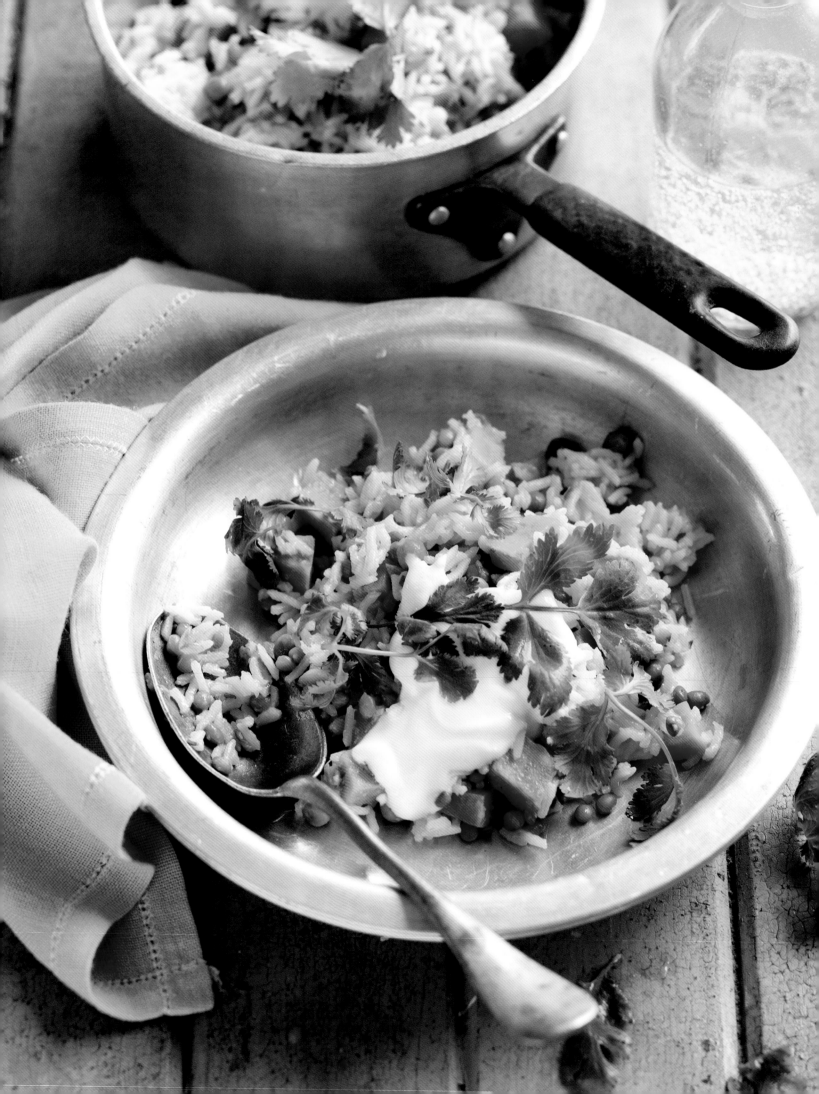

kitchari

PREP + COOK TIME 40 MINUTES ◆ **SERVES** 2

1 tablespoon olive oil

2 teaspoons grated fresh ginger

2 cloves garlic, crushed

3 whole cloves

½ teaspoon cumin seeds

½ fresh long green chilli,
sliced finely

1 fresh bay leaf

½ small kumara (orange sweet
potato) (125g), peeled, cut into
1cm (½-inch) pieces

¼ cup (30g) frozen peas

½ cup (100g) basmati rice

1½ cups (375ml) water

½ teaspoon salt-reduced
chicken stock powder

½ cup (85g) rinsed, drained
canned brown lentils

¼ cup (70g) low-fat plain yoghurt

2 tablespoons fresh coriander
leaves (cilantro)

Kitchari, an ancient Indian dish, is often eaten to detoxify the body, and is believed to aid digestion. It is based on the practise of Ayurveda, which focuses on the body's overall balance and harmony.

1 Heat oil in a medium saucepan over low heat; cook ginger, garlic, cloves, seeds, chilli and bay leaf, stirring occasionally, for 1 minute or until fragrant.

2 Stir kumara, peas, rice, the water and stock powder into pan. Shake the pan to evenly settle the rice; bring to the boil. Reduce heat; cover, simmer, without stirring, for 15 minutes.

3 Remove from heat; stand, covered, for 10 minutes, then fold through the lentils. Serve rice mixture topped with yoghurt and coriander.

TIP Kitchari can be served as a breakfast dish with a poached egg and wholemeal flatbread.

mushroom, cavolo nero and quinoa risotto

PREP + COOK TIME 40 MINUTES ◆ SERVES 2

10g (½ ounce) dried porcini mushrooms

½ cup (125ml) boiling water

1 tablespoon olive oil

1 small brown onion (80g), chopped finely

1 flat mushroom (80g), chopped coarsely

100g (3 ounces) swiss brown mushrooms, sliced thinly

2 cloves garlic, crushed

½ cup quinoa (100g), rinsed, drained

2½ cups (625ml) salt-reduced vegetable stock

1 sprig fresh thyme

100g (3 ounces) cavolo nero, sliced thinly

⅓ cup (25g) finely grated parmesan

1   Place porcini mushrooms in a heatproof bowl; cover with the boiling water. Stand for 5 minutes.

2   Meanwhile, heat oil in a medium frying pan over medium heat; cook onion, stirring, for 3 minutes or until soft. Add flat and swiss brown mushrooms; cook, stirring, for 3 minutes or until browned and tender. Add garlic; cook, stirring, for 1 minute or until fragrant.

3   Stir in quinoa, stock and thyme. Remove porcini mushrooms from water (reserve the soaking liquid); chop coarsely. Add mushrooms and soaking liquid to pan. Bring to the boil; simmer, uncovered for 20 minutes until liquid is absorbed and quinoa is tender. Discard thyme.

4   Add cavolo nero; stir until wilted. Remove pan from heat; stir through half the parmesan.

5   Serve risotto topped with remaining parmesan.

TIP Cavolo nero is also known as tuscan cabbage; it is highly nutritious, and is also great to use in soups, salads and stir-fries.

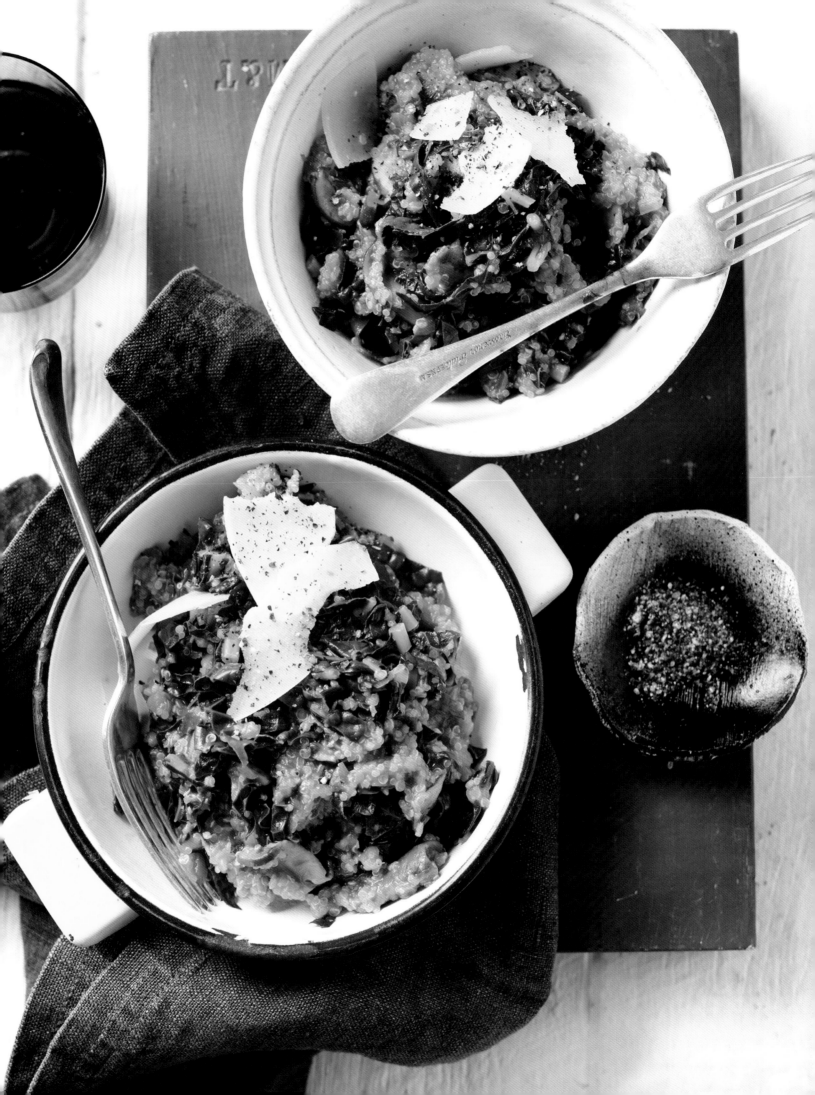

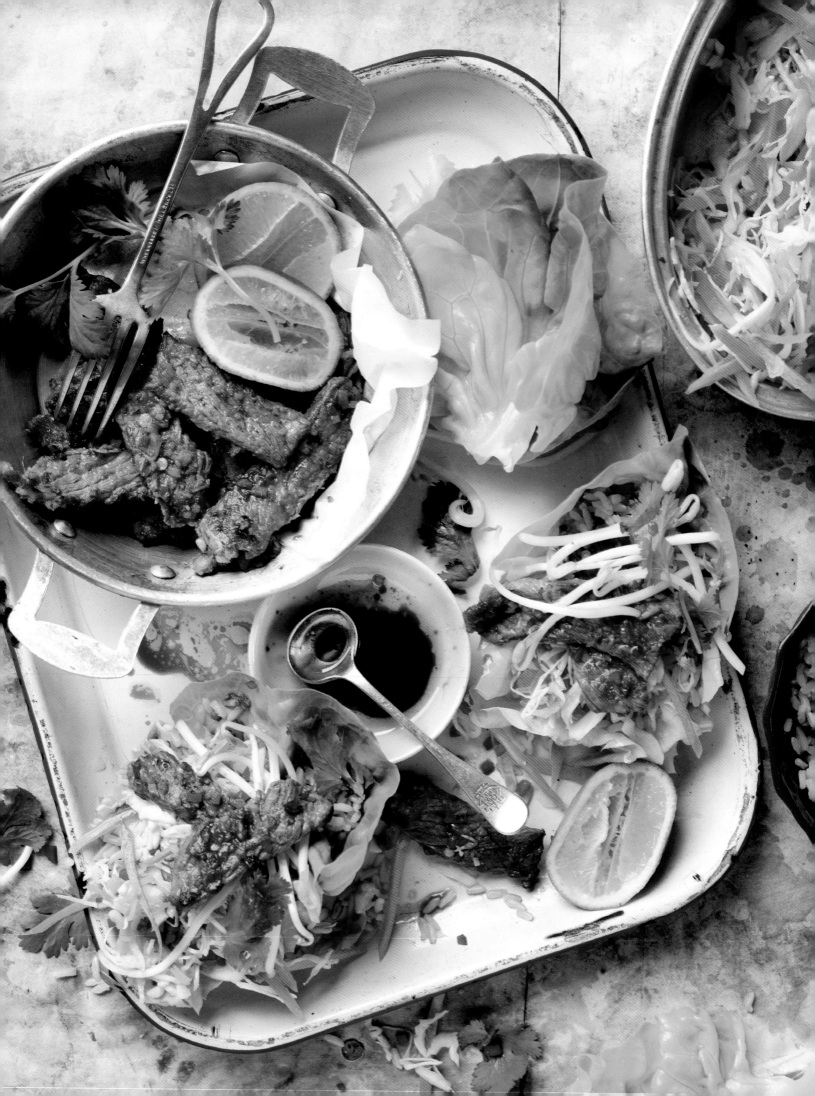

korean beef lettuce cups with pickled vegetables

PREP + COOK TIME 40 MINUTES (+ REFRIGERATION) ◆ SERVES 2

1 fresh long red chilli, chopped coarsely

1 tablespoon coarsely chopped lemon grass

2 cloves garlic, halved

2 teaspoons finely chopped fresh ginger

1 tablespoon water

3 teaspoons reduced-salt soy sauce

150g (4½ ounces) lean beef sirloin steak, trimmed, thinly sliced

½ cup (100g) low-GI brown rice (doongara)

2 teaspoons rice bran oil

6 large butter lettuce leaves (50g)

1 teaspoon sesame oil

¼ cup firmly packed fresh coriander leaves (cilantro)

½ cup (40g) bean sprouts, trimmed

PICKLED CABBAGE

1 fresh long red chilli, chopped finely

1 small carrot (70g), cut into matchsticks

1½ cups (120g) shredded green cabbage

2 teaspoons caster (superfine) sugar

1 tablespoon rice wine vinegar

1 Blend or process chilli, lemon grass, garlic, ginger, the water and half the sauce until smooth. Combine chilli mixture and beef in a small bowl. Cover; refrigerate for 30 minutes.

2 Cook rice in a medium saucepan of boiling water, stirring occasionally, for 25 minutes or until tender; drain well.

3 Meanwhile, make pickled cabbage.

4 Heat rice bran oil in a wok over high heat; cook beef, in batches, for 30 seconds or until browned all over.

5 Spoon rice into lettuce leaves, top with some of the pickled cabbage, then some of the beef. Combine remaining sauce and sesame oil; drizzle over beef. Sprinkle with coriander and sprouts.

PICKLED CABBAGE Combine ingredients in a large bowl. Stand for 30 minutes to soften and develop the flavours.

TIPS Freeze beef slightly to make it easier to cut into thin slices. Remove seeds from chilli for a milder heat.

NUTRITIONAL COUNT PER SERVING

● 10.2g total fat
● 2.4g saturated fat
● 1509kJ (360 cal)
● 27g carbohydrate
● 32.3g protein
● 19.3g fibre
● 172mg sodium
● low GI

barbecued steak with white bean puree and chimichurri

PREP + COOK TIME 2 HOURS (+ STANDING) ◆ **SERVES** 2

½ **cup dried cannellini beans**

4 cloves garlic, peeled

1½ **tablespoons lemon juice**

¼ **cup (60ml) water**

150g (4½ ounces) lean beef skirt steak, trimmed

1 teaspoon rice bran oil

1 tablespoon coarsely chopped fresh oregano

2 cups (230g) watercress sprigs

½ **small red onion (50g), sliced thinly**

CHIMICHURRI

1¼ **cups fresh flat-leaf parsley leaves, chopped finely**

¼ **cup fresh oregano leaves, chopped finely**

1 clove garlic, crushed

¼ **teaspoon chilli flakes**

1 tablespoon red wine vinegar

2 teaspoons dijon mustard

1 teaspoon rice bran oil

1 Place beans in a large bowl; cover with cold water. Stand overnight. Drain well.

2 Cook beans and garlic in a large saucepan of boiling water for 1½ hours or until very tender. Drain well.

3 Blend or process beans, garlic, juice and the water until smooth. Season with pepper to taste. Transfer to a small bowl, cover to keep warm.

4 Meanwhile, make chimichurri.

5 Drizzle steaks with oil, sprinkle with oregano. Heat a grill pan (or grill or barbecue) over medium high heat; cook beef for 3 minutes each side for medium or until cooked as desired. Transfer to a plate; cover, stand for 10 minutes.

6 Slice beef; serve with bean puree, chimichurri and combined watercress and onion.

CHIMICHURRI Combine ingredients in a small bowl; mix well. Season with pepper to taste.

TIPS You will need 1½ cups cooked beans. You can use 60g (2 ounces) baby rocket leaves (arugula) instead of watercress, if you like.

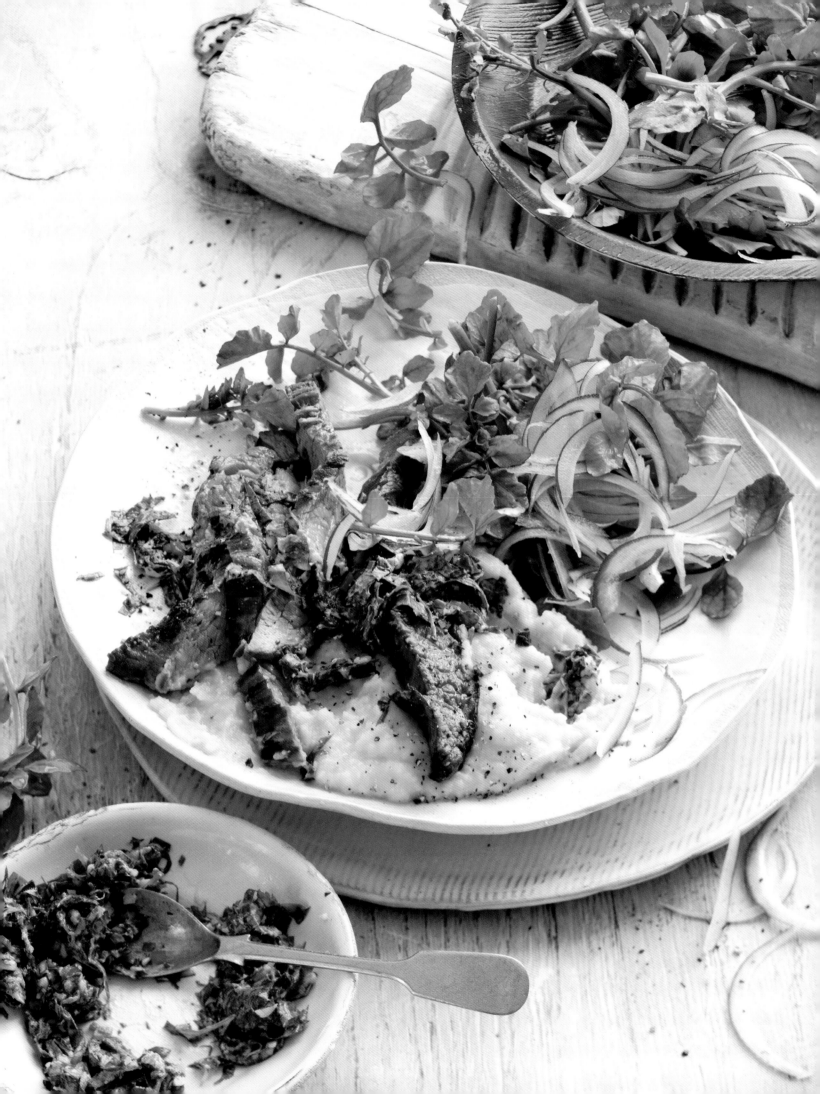

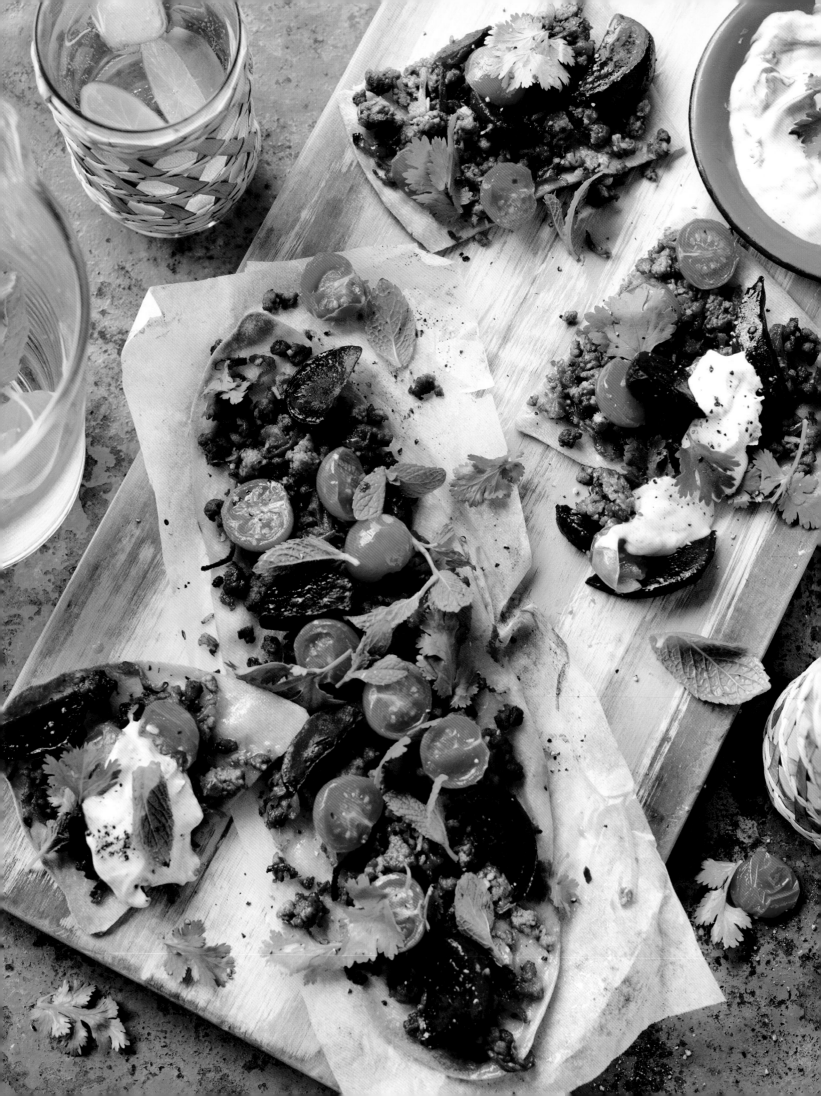

beetroot & lamb flatbreads with tahini yoghurt

PREP + COOK TIME 50 MINUTES (+ STANDING) ◆ SERVES 2

¼ cup (40g) wholemeal plain (all-purpose) flour

½ cup (75g) plain (all-purpose) flour

⅓ cup (80ml) water, approximately

2 teaspoons rice bran oil

1 small red onion (100g), sliced thinly

100g (3 ounces) lean minced (ground) lamb

3 cloves garlic, crushed

2 teaspoons ground cumin

¼ teaspoon chilli flakes

100g (3 ounces) canned drained beetroot (beet) wedges

125g (4 ounces) cherry tomatoes, halved

2 tablespoons each fresh mint and coriander (cilantro) leaves

TAHINI YOGHURT

¼ cup (70g) no-fat plain yoghurt

2 teaspoons tahini (sesame seed paste)

1 clove garlic, crushed

2 teaspoons lemon juice

2 teaspoons coarsely chopped fresh coriander (cilantro)

2 teaspoons coarsely chopped fresh mint

½ teaspoon ground cumin

2 teaspoons water

1 Combine sifted flours in a large bowl. Add enough of the water to mix to a soft dough. Turn out onto a lightly floured surface. Knead gently for 1 minute or until smooth. Divide dough into two portions. Cover, stand for 30 minutes.

2 Heat oil in a large non-stick frying pan over medium-low heat; cook onion, stirring, for 5 minutes or until soft. Add mince; cook, stirring, over high heat, for 5 minutes or until browned. Add garlic, cumin and chilli; cook, stirring, for 1 minute or until fragrant. Season with pepper to taste.

3 Preheat oven to 220°C/425°F. Roll one piece of dough between two pieces of baking paper to make a 30cm (12-inch) oval. Discard top sheet of paper. Transfer bottom sheet of baking paper and dough onto a large baking tray. Top with half the lamb mixture, half the beetroot and half the tomato. Repeat with remaining dough, lamb, beetroot and tomato to make two flatbreads.

4 Bake for 15 minutes, swapping trays halfway through cooking time, or until bases are browned and crisp.

5 Meanwhile, make tahini yoghurt.

6 Drizzle flatbreads with tahini yoghurt; sprinkle with mint and coriander leaves, to serve.

TAHINI YOGHURT Combine ingredients in a small bowl; season with pepper.

cutlets with smashed potatoes and brussels sprouts salad

PREP + COOK TIME 1 HOUR ◆ SERVES 2

2 medium potatoes (400g)

2 teaspoons rice bran oil

1 tablespoon fennel seeds

1 tablespoon fresh rosemary leaves

6 french-trimmed lamb cutlets (300g)

1 tablespoon honey

1 tablespoon lemon juice

¼ cup (60ml) water

1½ cups shredded cavolo nero (tuscan cabbage) (200g)

12 brussels sprouts (370g), sliced finely

1 tablespoon balsamic vinegar

1   Preheat oven to 220°C/425°F. Line an oven tray with baking paper.

2   Cook potatoes in a small saucepan of boiling water for 10 minutes or until tender; drain. Place potatoes on oven tray; crush with a potato masher. Drizzle with half the oil, sprinkle with half the fennel seeds and half the rosemary. Season with ground black pepper. Bake for 30 minutes or until browned and crisp.

3   Meanwhile, coat lamb in remaining oil; sprinkle with remaining fennel seeds and rosemary. Heat an oiled grill plate (or grill or barbecue) over medium-high heat; cook cutlets for 3 minutes each side or until browned and tender. Transfer to a plate; drizzle with honey and half the juice. Cover; stand for 5 minutes.

4   Heat a large frying pan over high heat, add the water, cavolo nero and sprouts; cook, stirring, for 2 minutes or until vegetables are just tender. Toss through vinegar and the remaining juice.

5   Serve cutlets and potatoes with vegetables.

TIPS Use a mandoline or a V-slicer to thinly slice the brussels sprouts. If brussels sprouts are not in season, try making the salad with thinly sliced broccoli or shredded cabbage. Silver beet or kale can be substituted for cavolo nero.

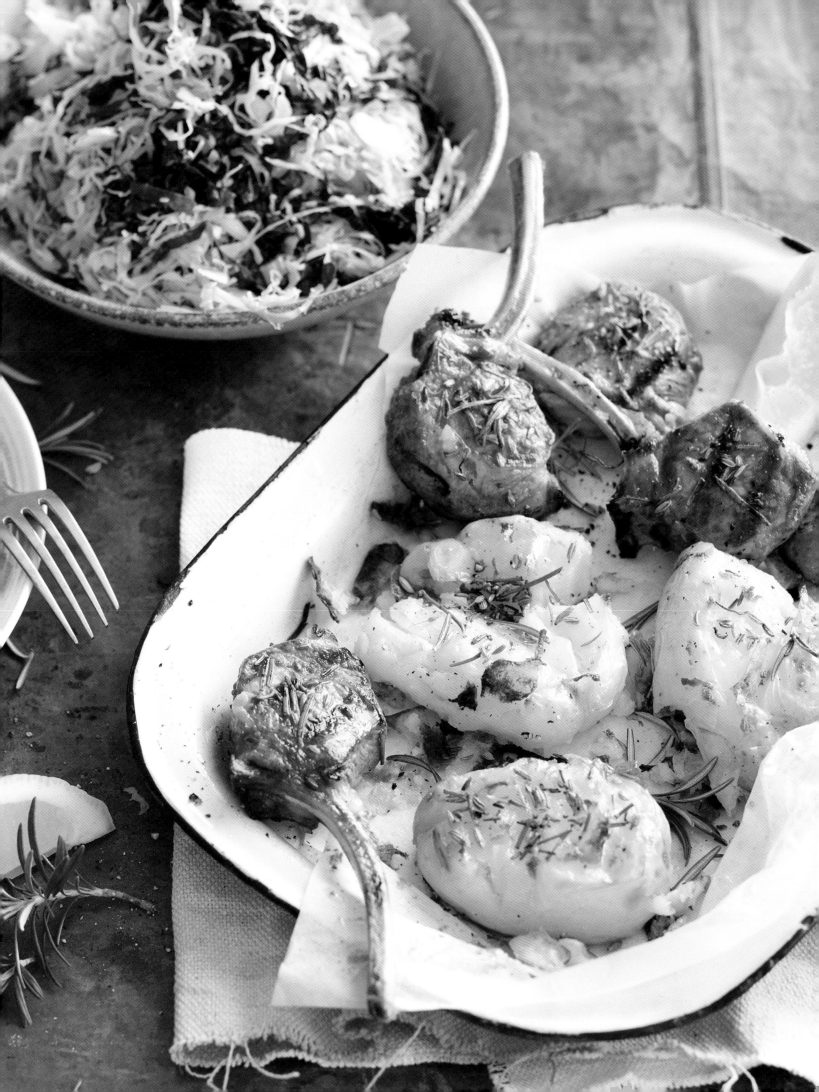

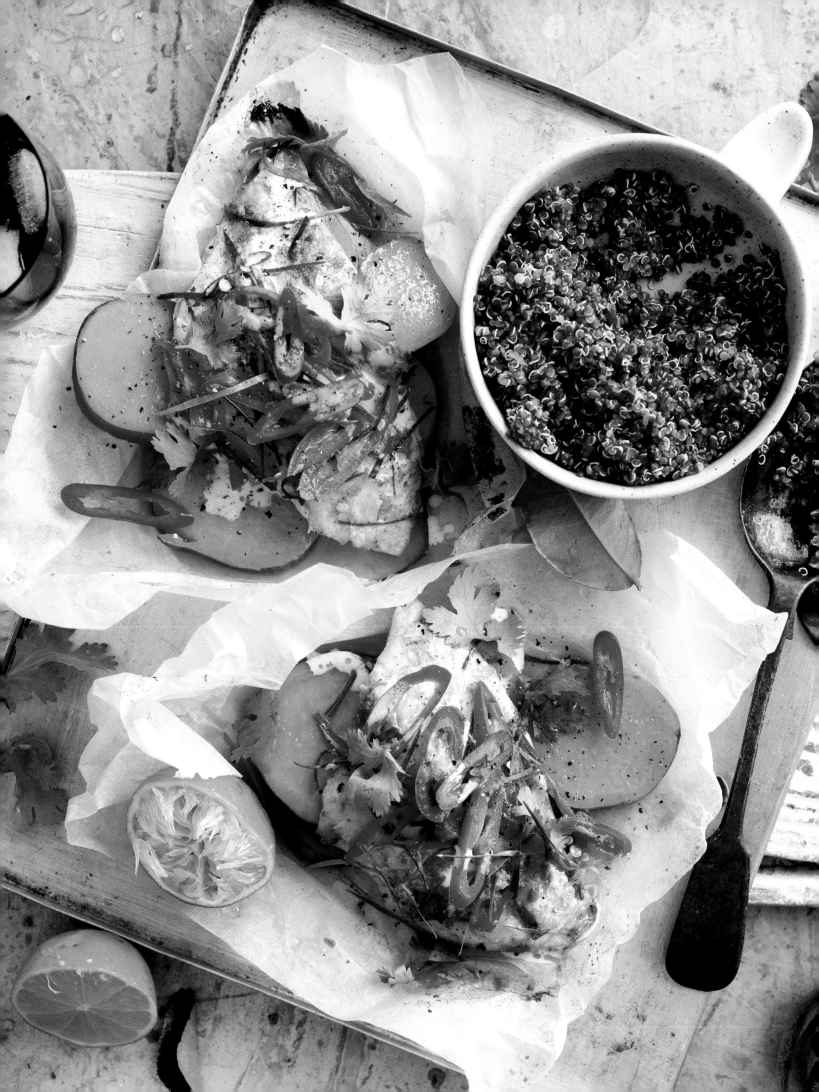

NUTRITIONAL COUNT PER SERVING

● 7g total fat   ● 47g protein
● 1.7g saturated fat   ● 5.2g fibre
● 1660kJ (396 cal)   ● 432mg sodium;
● 33.2g carbohydrate   ● low GI

kaffir lime and red curry fish parcels

PREP + COOK TIME 30 MINUTES (+ REFRIGERATION) ◆ **SERVES** 2

2 teaspoons red curry paste

4 shredded kaffir lime leaves

2 coriander roots (cilantro) with 1cm (½-inch) of stem, bruised

1 fresh long red chilli, sliced finely

2 x 200g (7 ounces) firm boneless white fish fillets, skin on

1 small kumara (orange sweet potato) (250g), cut into 1cm (½-inch) thick slices

2 teaspoons lime juice

2 tablespoons red quinoa

2 teaspoons light coconut milk

2 tablespoons fresh coriander (cilantro) leaves

1 Combine paste, lime leaves, coriander roots and stems, and half the chilli in a small bowl. Rub fish fillets with mixture; cover, refrigerate for 1 hour or overnight.

2 Preheat oven to 220°C/425°F.

3 Place kumara in a small saucepan, cover with cold water; bring to the boil, simmer, uncovered, for 5 minutes or until just tender, drain.

4 Cut two pieces of foil 50cm x 30cm (19-inches x 12-inches); place on work surface, shiny-side up. Lay two 48cm x 30cm (18-inch x 12-inch) pieces of baking paper over foil.

5 Divide kumara and fish mixture between paper, drizzle with juice. Fold foil over to completely enclose fish and kumara.

6 Place fish parcels on a large baking tray. Bake parcels for 15 minutes or until fish is cooked through. Discard coriander roots and stems.

7 Meanwhile, rinse and drain quinoa well. Place in a small saucepan, cover with water; bring to the boil, boil for 10 minutes or until tender, drain.

8 Serve fish with quinoa; top with coconut milk, remaining chilli and coriander leaves.

TIPS We used snapper for this recipe. The parcels can be made to the end of step 5 and refrigerated for up to 1 day in advance. Heat reflects off the shiny side of aluminium foil, so having the shiny side facing into the parcel ensures maximum heat penetrating the fish.

chicken and pumpkin pot pies

PREP + COOK TIME 45 MINUTES ◆ SERVES 2

250g (8 ounces) chicken breast fillet

450g (14½ ounces) butternut pumpkin, chopped coarsely

1 small leek (200g), sliced thinly

1 clove garlic, crushed

¼ teaspoon thyme leaves

¼ cup (60ml) water

1 teaspoon plain (all-purpose) flour

2 sheets fillo pastry

1 egg white, beaten lightly

1 teaspoon coarsely chopped pepitas

30g (1 ounce) firmly packed small beetroot leaves

1 teaspoon lemon juice

1 Place chicken in a medium saucepan; cover with cold water. Bring to the boil; reduce heat, simmer, uncovered, for 10 minutes or until chicken is cooked through. Drain chicken reserving ½ cup of the poaching liquid. Shred chicken.

2 Meanwhile, boil, steam or microwave pumpkin until tender; mash coarsely.

3 Preheat oven to 200°C/400°F.

4 Cook leek, garlic, thyme and the water in a medium saucepan over medium heat, stirring occasionally, for 5 minutes or until leek is tender. Add flour; cook, stirring, for 2 minutes or until slightly thickened. Add chicken, reserved poaching liquid and pumpkin, bring to the boil, stirring, for 2 minutes or until thickened slightly. Season with pepper to taste.

5 Brush pastry sheets with egg white, folding in half three times to make a square. Brush edges of two 1-cup (250ml) heatproof ramekins with egg white. Divide chicken mixture between ramekins, top with pastry squares turning edges of pastry upwards. Brush tops with egg white. Using a small sharp knife, make a hole in the centre of each pie; sprinkle with pepitas. Bake pies for 25 minutes or until pastry is browned lightly.

6 Combine beetroot leaves and juice in a small bowl, season with pepper to taste. Serve hot pies with beetroot leaves.

TIP Filling can be prepared up to two days ahead; store, covered, in the fridge.

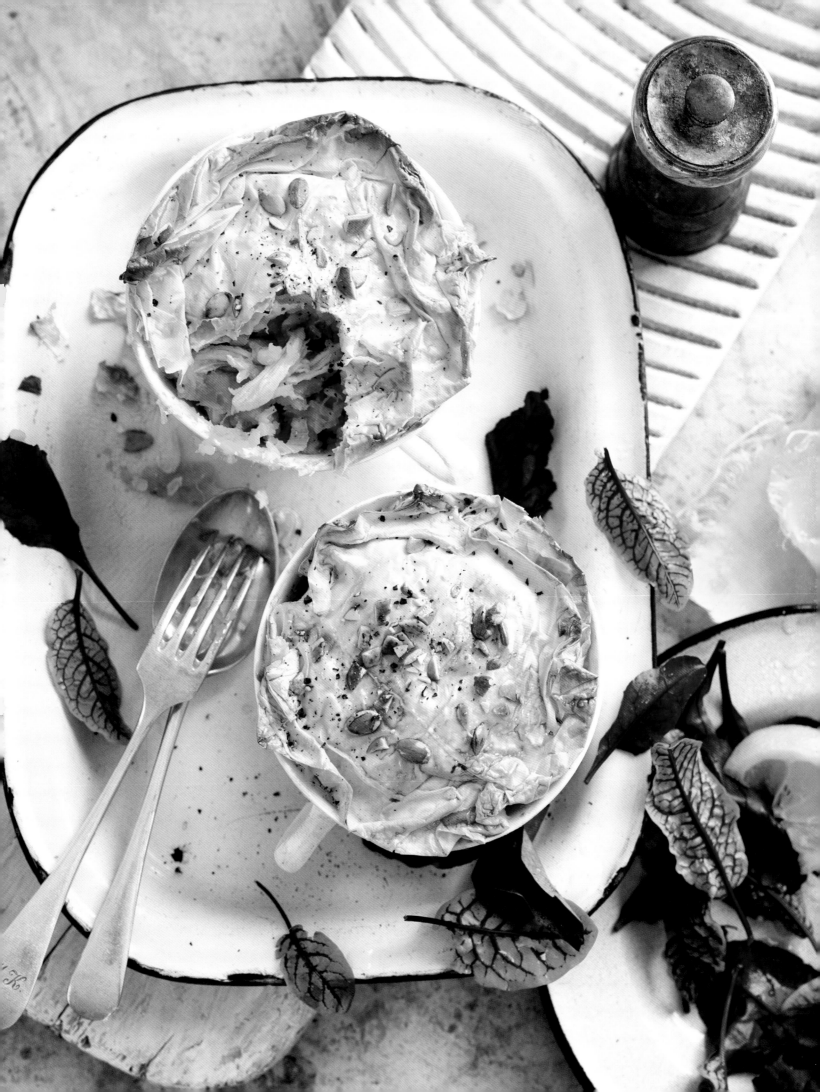

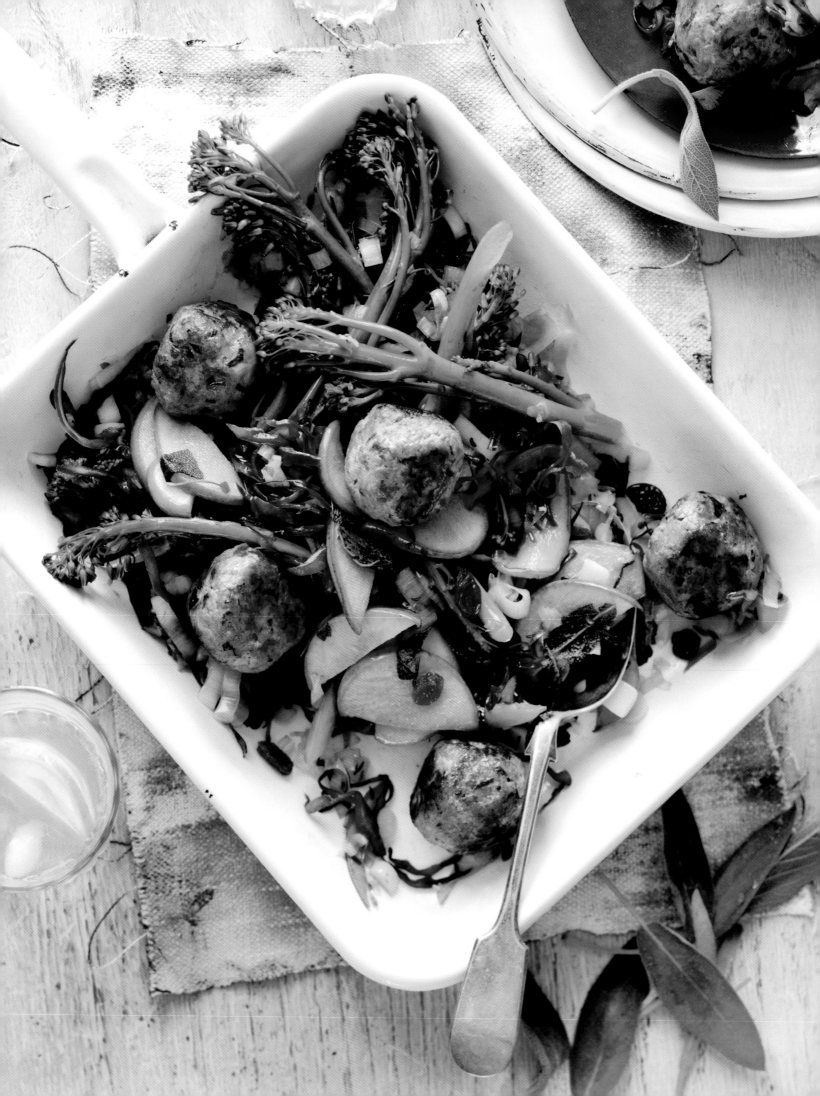

pork and sage meatballs with cabbage and pear

PREP + COOK TIME 40 MINUTES (+ REFRIGERATION) ◆ SERVES 2

175g (5½ ounces) lean minced (ground) pork

⅓ cup (25g) fresh multigrain breadcrumbs

1 small egg white

1 teaspoon finely grated lemon rind

½ teaspoon allspice

1 small brown onion (80g), grated coarsely

1 tablespoon chopped fresh sage leaves

2 tablespoons chopped fresh flat-leaf parsley leaves

2 teaspoons rice bran oil

1 small leek (200g), halved, sliced thinly

1 medium pear (230g), sliced thinly

85g (3 ounces) broccolini, trimmed

2 cups (160g) finely shredded red cabbage

½ teaspoon caraway seeds

1 tablespoon small sage leaves

1 tablespoon sultanas

1 Combine pork, breadcrumbs, egg white, rind, allspice, onion, chopped sage and parsley in a medium bowl; mix well. Form mixture into six balls. Place on a tray; cover, refrigerate for 30 minutes to firm.

2 Heat half the oil in a large non-stick frying pan over low heat; cook meatballs, turning, for 8 minutes or until browned and cooked through. Transfer to a clean tray; cover with foil to keep warm.

3 Heat remaining oil in a large saucepan over medium-high heat; cook leek, stirring, for 3 minutes. Add pear and broccolini; cook, turning occasionally, for 3 minutes. Add cabbage, caraway, sage leaves and sultanas; cook, stirring, for 3 minutes or until just tender.

4 Serve vegetables with meatballs.

TIPS You could double the meatball recipe to serve 4 or freeze a batch for another meal. Meatballs will freeze for up to 3 months; thaw overnight in the fridge before cooking.

pasta with spinach, mushrooms & almonds

PREP + COOK TIME 30 MINUTES ◆ **SERVES** 2

200g (6½ ounces) wholegrain spaghetti

3 teaspoons rice bran oil

300g (10 ounces) swiss brown mushrooms, sliced

300g (10 ounces) portobello mushrooms, sliced

1 shallot (25g), chopped coarsely

1 clove garlic, chopped coarsely

1 tablespoon firmly packed fresh flat-leaf parsley

¼ cup (40g) coarsely chopped unsalted, roasted almonds

100g (3 ounces) baby spinach leaves

¼ cup (20g) flaked pecorino cheese

1 Cook pasta in a large saucepan of boiling water until tender; reserve ½ cup of the liquid, drain pasta.

2 Meanwhile, heat oil in a large frying pan over high heat; cook mushrooms and shallot, stirring occasionally, for 5 minutes or until mushrooms are lightly golden and shallot is tender. Add garlic and parsley; cook, stirring, for 1 minute or until garlic is fragrant. Season to taste with black pepper.

3 Reduce heat to low; toss warm pasta, nuts and spinach through mushroom mixture. Add enough reserved pasta water to lightly coat the pasta. Serve topped with cheese.

TIPS You can use 600g (1¼ ounces) of your favourite variety of mushrooms; button and cap mushrooms will work well. If you don't have a large frying pan, cook the mushrooms in batches to prevent them stewing.

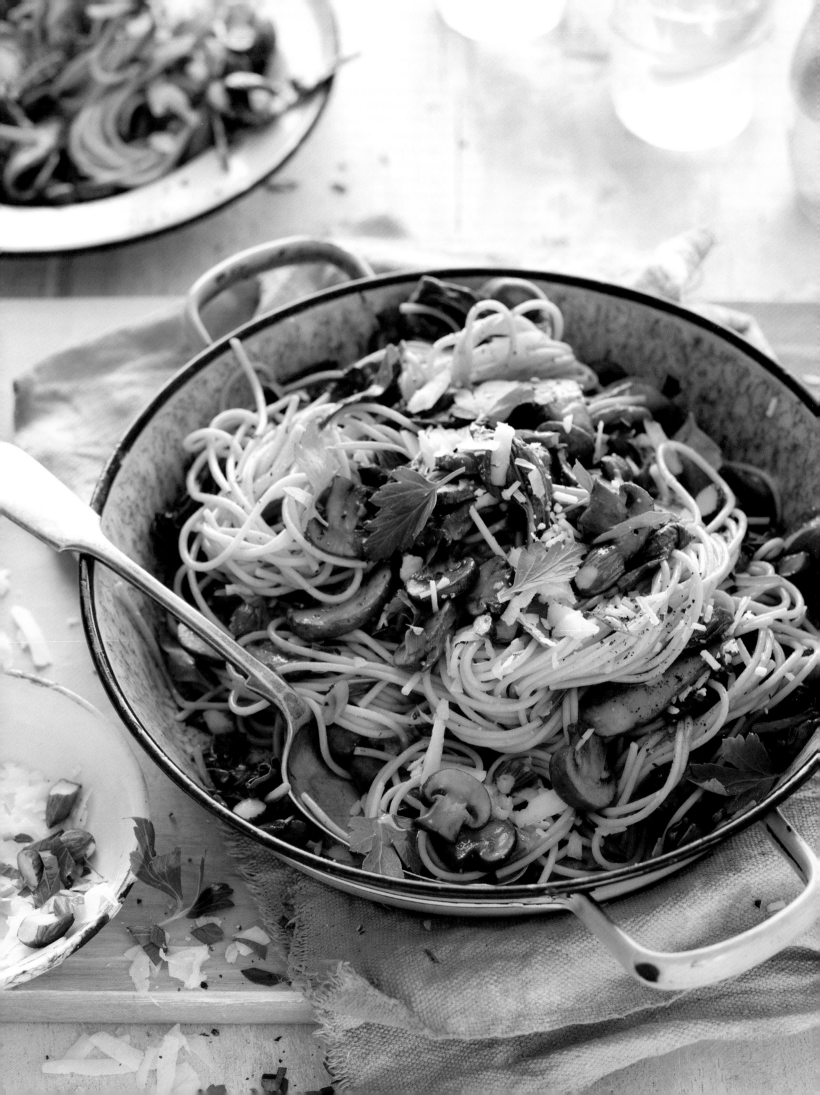

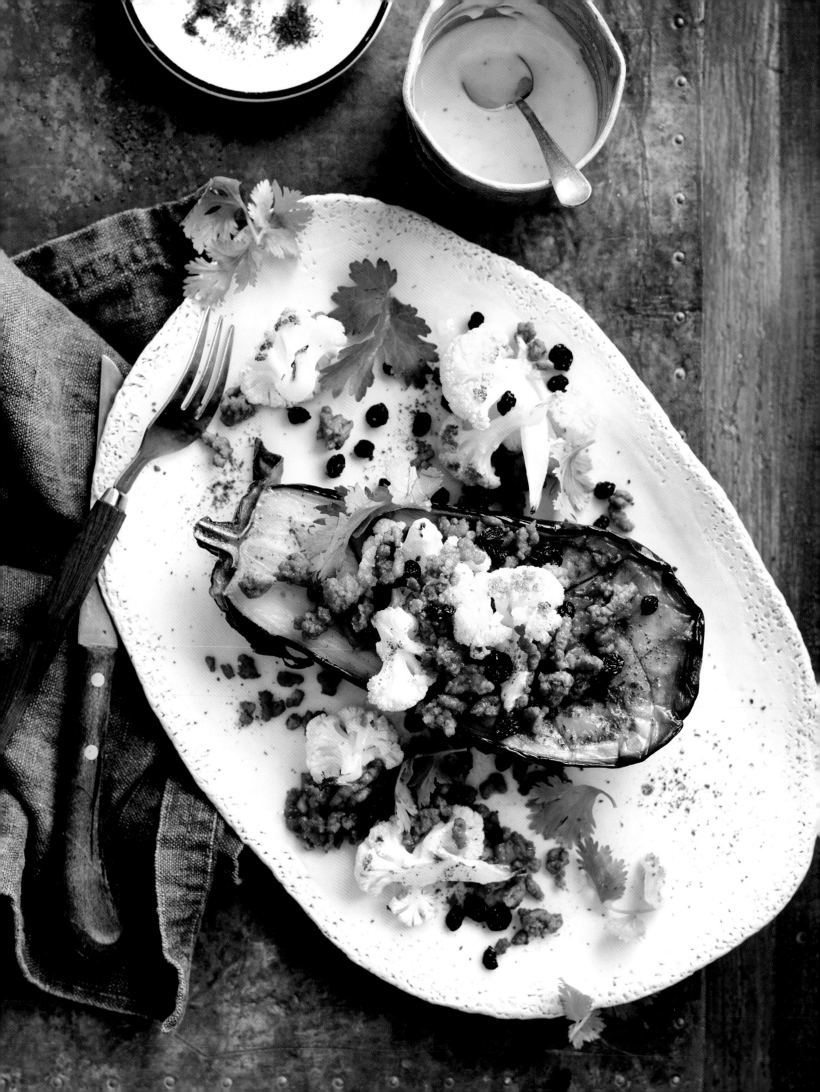

roasted eggplant with spiced lamb

PREP + COOK TIME 45 MINUTES ◆ **SERVES** 2

1 large eggplant (500g), halved lengthways

2 teaspoons olive oil

350g (11 ounces) cauliflower, chopped coarsely

150g (4½ ounces) lean minced (ground) lamb

1 teaspoon each ground cumin and coriander

2 tablespoons water

2 teaspoons pomegranate molasses

½ cup (140g) fat-free natural yoghurt

2 teaspoons lemon juice

1 clove garlic, crushed

2 tablespoons currants

½ cup fresh coriander leaves (cilantro)

½ teaspoon sumac

1 Preheat oven to 200°C/400°F. Line a large oven tray with baking paper.

2 Using a sharp knife, score the eggplant flesh diagonally. Drizzle with half the oil. Place flesh-side down on tray. Roast for 10 minutes. Add cauliflower to tray; drizzle with remaining oil. Roast a further 30 minutes or until tender.

3 Meanwhile, heat a medium oiled non-stick frying pan over high heat; cook lamb, spices and the water, stirring, until browned. Add pomegranate molasses. Remove from heat.

4 Combine yoghurt, juice and garlic in a small bowl.

5 Serve eggplant topped with cauliflower, lamb, currants and coriander. Spoon over yoghurt mixture and sprinkle with sumac.

TIP Sumac is a spice made from ground berries and has a lemony flavour. It is available from supermarkets and spice shops.

lamb with heirloom tomato and almond salad

PREP + COOK TIME 15 MINUTES ◆ SERVES 2

½ cup (110g) risoni pasta

4 french-trimmed lamb cutlets (200g)

1 clove garlic, crushed

2 teaspoons finely chopped fresh rosemary leaves

2 teaspoons extra virgin olive oil

400g (12½ ounces) heirloom tomatoes, sliced

2 tablespoons flaked almonds, toasted

½ cup loosely packed fresh basil leaves

40g (1½ ounce) buffalo mozzarella, torn

1 tablespoon red wine vinegar

2 teaspoons extra virgin olive oil, extra

1 Cook pasta in a large saucepan of boiling water until tender; drain.

2 Meanwhile, combine lamb with garlic, rosemary and oil in a medium bowl. Cook lamb on a heated grill plate (or grill or barbecue) for 2 minutes each side or until cooked as desired.

3 Toss pasta with tomato, nuts, basil and cheese in a large bowl. Drizzle with vinegar and extra oil. Serve salad topped with lamb.

TIP If you can't find buffalo mozzarella, use bocconcini.

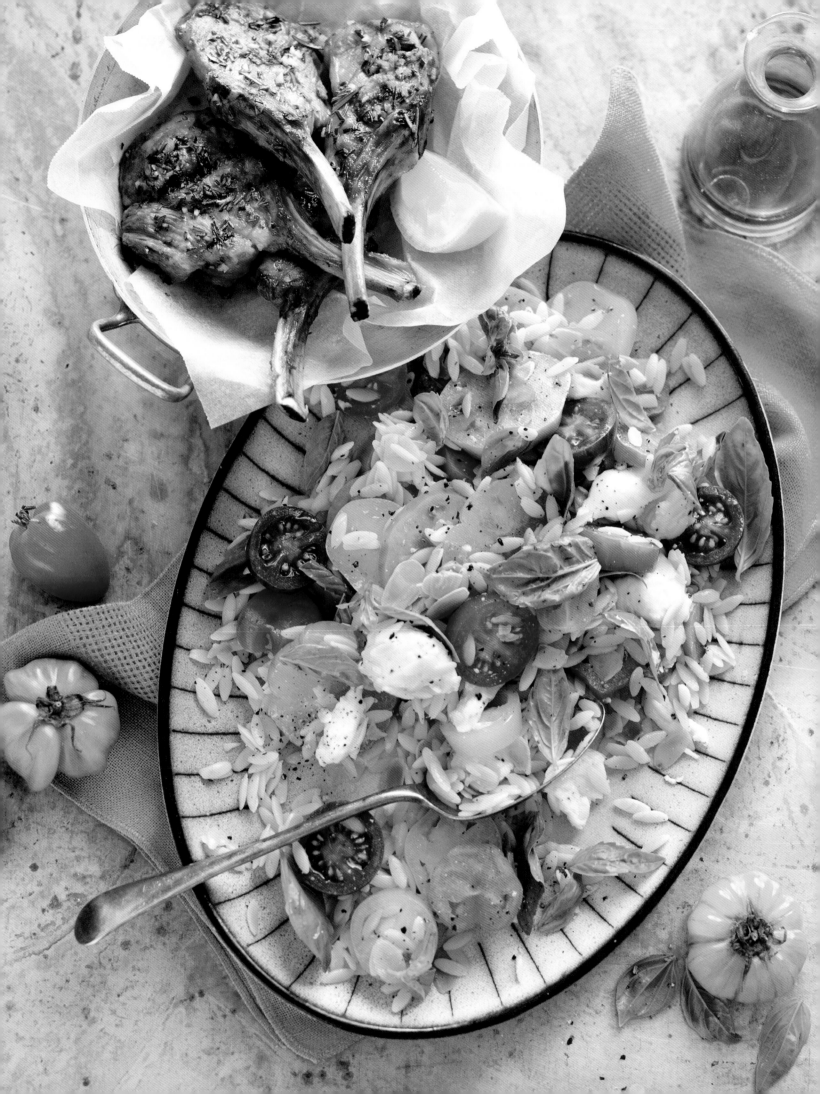

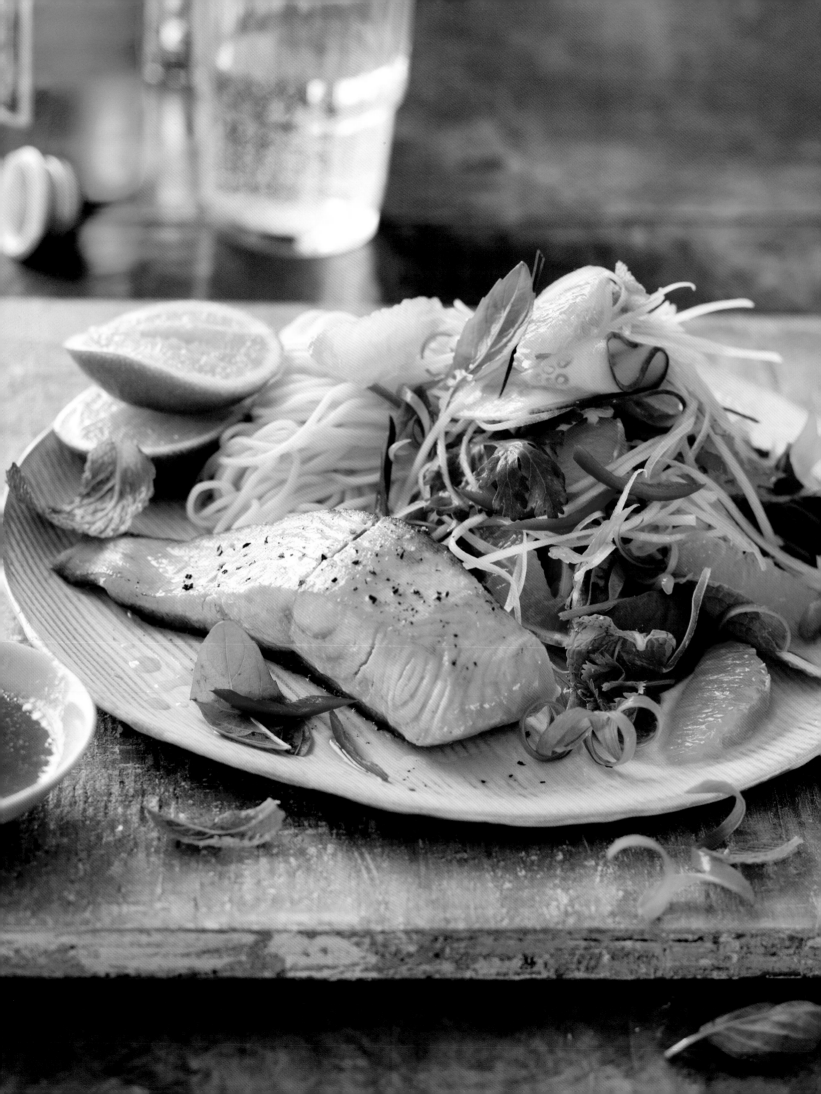

salmon with green papaya & pink grapefruit salad

PREP + COOK TIME 35 MINUTES ◆ SERVES 2

100g (3 ounces) dry egg noodles

1 lebanese cucumber (130g), cut into ribbons

70g (2½ ounces) shredded green papaya

3 shallots (75g), sliced finely

1 small ruby grapefruit (350g), peeled, segmented

1 fresh long red chilli, chopped finely

½ cup loosely packed fresh mint leaves

½ cup loosely packed fresh coriander (cilantro) leaves

½ cup loosely packed fresh thai basil leaves

1 tablespoon shredded kaffir lime leaves

2 tablespoons lime juice

1 teaspoon fish sauce

1 tablespoon brown sugar

2 teaspoons rice bran oil

200g (6½ ounces) skinless salmon fillet, trimmed, halved lengthways

1 Cook noodles according to packet directions. Drain, rinse under cold water.

2 Meanwhile, combine cucumber, papaya, shallot, grapefruit, chilli, herbs and lime leaves in a large bowl. Drizzle with combined juice, sauce and sugar; toss gently to combine.

3 Heat oil in a medium non-stick frying pan over high heat; cook fish for 2 minutes each side or until just cooked through.

4 Serve fish with salad and noodles.

TIPS Swap the salmon for tuna steaks if you like. If papaya is unavailable you could use green mango. Remove the seeds from the chilli to reduce the heat.

wholegrain pizza marinara

PREP + COOK TIME 45 MINUTES (+ REFRIGERATION & STANDING) ◆ **SERVES** 2

1 fresh long red chilli, chopped finely

1 clove garlic, crushed

1 teaspoon finely grated lemon rind

1 tablespoon coarsely chopped fresh flat-leaf parsley

1 tablespoon rice bran oil

4 peeled medium king prawns (shrimp) (90g)

2 whole cleaned baby octopus (180g), halved lengthways

100g (3 ounces) cherry tomatoes, halved

25g (1 ounce) baby rocket leaves (arugula)

1 tablespoon fresh flat-leaf parsley leaves, extra

2 teaspoons lemon juice

DOUGH

1½ tablespoons cracked buckwheat

boiling water, to cover buckwheat

¼ cup (60ml) warm water

¼ teaspoon caster (superfine) sugar

½ teaspoon dried yeast

⅓ cup (55g) plain (all-purpose) flour

⅓ cup (60g) wholemeal plain (all-purpose) flour

1 Combine chilli, garlic, rind, parsley and oil in a small bowl, season with black pepper to taste. Divide garlic mixture in half; refrigerate one half of the mixture, covered. Combine remaining garlic mixture with prawns and octopus. Cover, refrigerate for 1 hour or overnight.

2 Make dough.

3 Meanwhile, preheat oven to 220°C/425°F. Lightly grease two large oven trays.

4 Bake pizza bases for 8 minutes or until partially cooked. Top with seafood mixture and tomato. Bake pizzas for a further 10 minutes or until bases are crisp and seafood is just cooked, drizzle with reserved garlic mixture.

5 Combine rocket, parsley and juice in a small bowl; season with pepper to taste.

6 Top pizzas with rocket mixture; serve immediately.

DOUGH Place buckwheat in a small heatproof bowl; cover with boiling water. Stand, covered for 30 minutes. Rinse under cold water; drain. Combine the warm water, sugar and yeast in a small jug, cover; stand in a warm place for 10 minutes or until frothy. Combine buckwheat and sifted flours in a medium bowl. Add yeast mixture; mix to a soft dough. Knead dough on a floured surface for 5 minutes or until smooth and elastic. Place dough in an oiled medium bowl. Cover; stand in a warm place for 45 minutes or until doubled in size. Halve dough. Roll each half into 15cm (6-inch) rounds; place on trays.

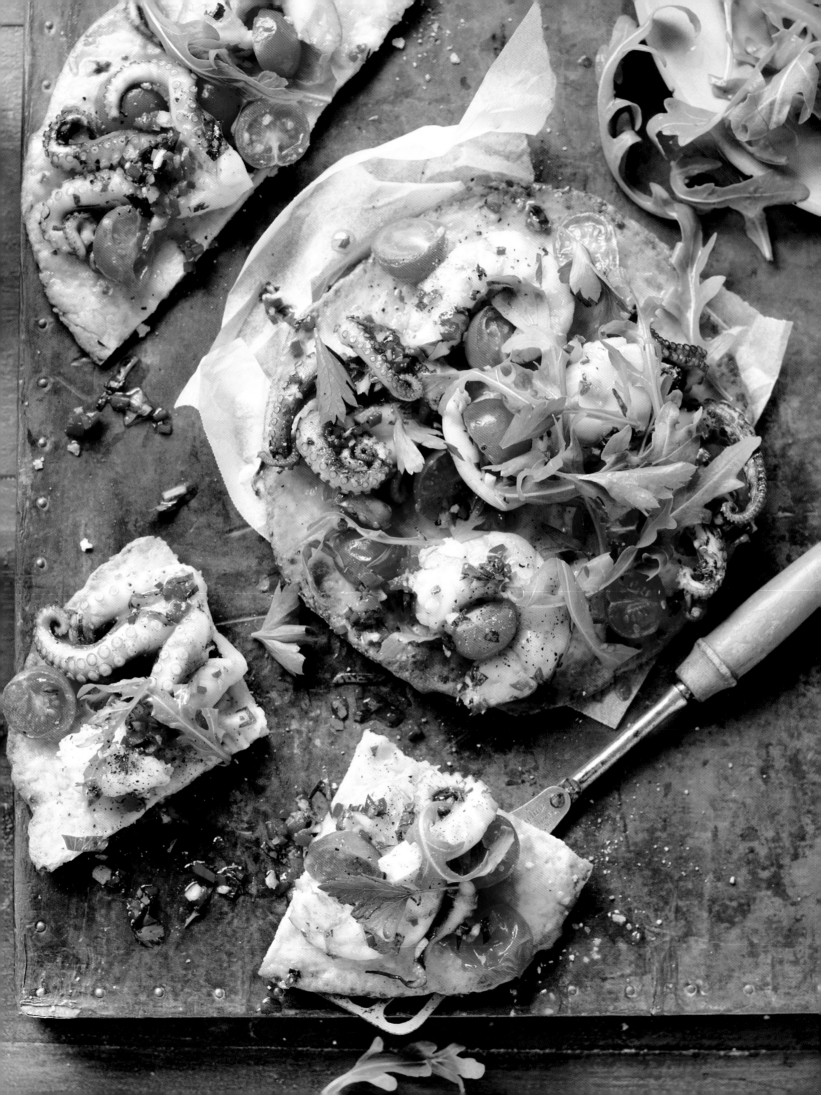

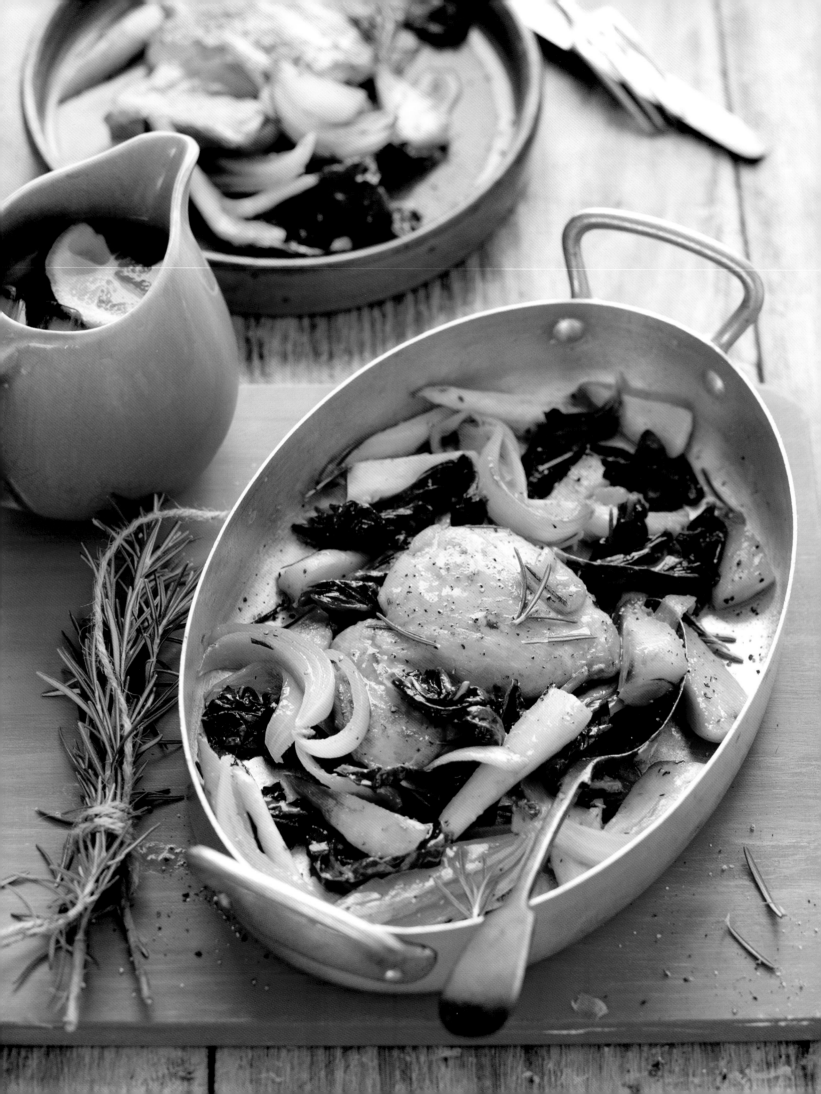

baked chicken with maple parsnips

PREP + COOK TIME 35 MINUTES ◆ SERVES 2

2 teaspoons rice bran oil

2 x 200g (6½ ounce) skinless chicken thigh cutlets

3 small parsnips (360g), chopped coarsely

1 medium brown onion (150g), cut into wedges

2 cloves garlic, sliced

2 sprigs fresh rosemary

1 tablespoon maple syrup

¼ cup (60ml) salt-reduced chicken stock

¼ cup (60ml) water

4 medium trimmed silver beet leaves (swiss chard) (140g)

1 Heat oil in a heavy-based saucepan over high heat; cook chicken for 2 minutes each side or until browned. Remove from pan; cover to keep warm.

2 Reduce heat to medium. Add parsnip, onion, garlic and rosemary to pan; cook for 5 minutes or until browned. Return chicken to pan with maple syrup, stock and the water. Bring to the boil; cover, reduce heat to low. Simmer for 15 minutes or until chicken is just cooked through. Stir in silver beet; cook for 2 minutes or until wilted.

TIP You could also use baby potatoes or carrots instead of the parsnips.

pork and tofu rice noodles

PREP + COOK TIME 25 MINUTES ◆ **SERVES** 2

125g (4 ounces) rice stick noodles

3 teaspoons rice bran oil

150g (4½ ounces) lean pork fillet, sliced thinly

150g (4½ ounces) firm tofu, drained, cut into 2.5cm (1-inch) cubes

2 cloves garlic, crushed

1 fresh small red thai (serrano) chilli, sliced thinly

1 small red onion (100g), cut into thin wedges

1 tablespoon water

1 medium yellow capsicum (bell pepper) (200g), sliced thinly

150g (4½ ounces) green beans, halved diagonally

150g (4½ ounces) oyster mushrooms, halved if large

2 tablespoons water, extra

1 tablespoon salt-reduced soy sauce

¼ cup loosely packed fresh coriander leaves (cilantro)

1 Place noodles in a medium heatproof bowl, cover with boiling water; stand until just tender, drain.

2 Meanwhile, heat 2 teaspoons of the oil in a wok over high heat; stir-fry pork for 3 minutes or until browned. Remove from wok; cover to keep warm.

3 Heat the remaining oil in wok over medium-high heat; stir-fry tofu, garlic, chilli, onion and the water for 3 minutes or until onion starts to soften. Add capsicum, beans and mushrooms to wok; stir-fry for 2 minutes. Add the extra water; stir-fry for 1 minute or until vegetables are just tender. Add sauce, pork and noodles; stir-fry until heated through.

4 Serve stir-fry topped with coriander.

TIP To make this recipe gluten-free, swap the soy sauce for 2 teaspoons of gluten-free tamari.

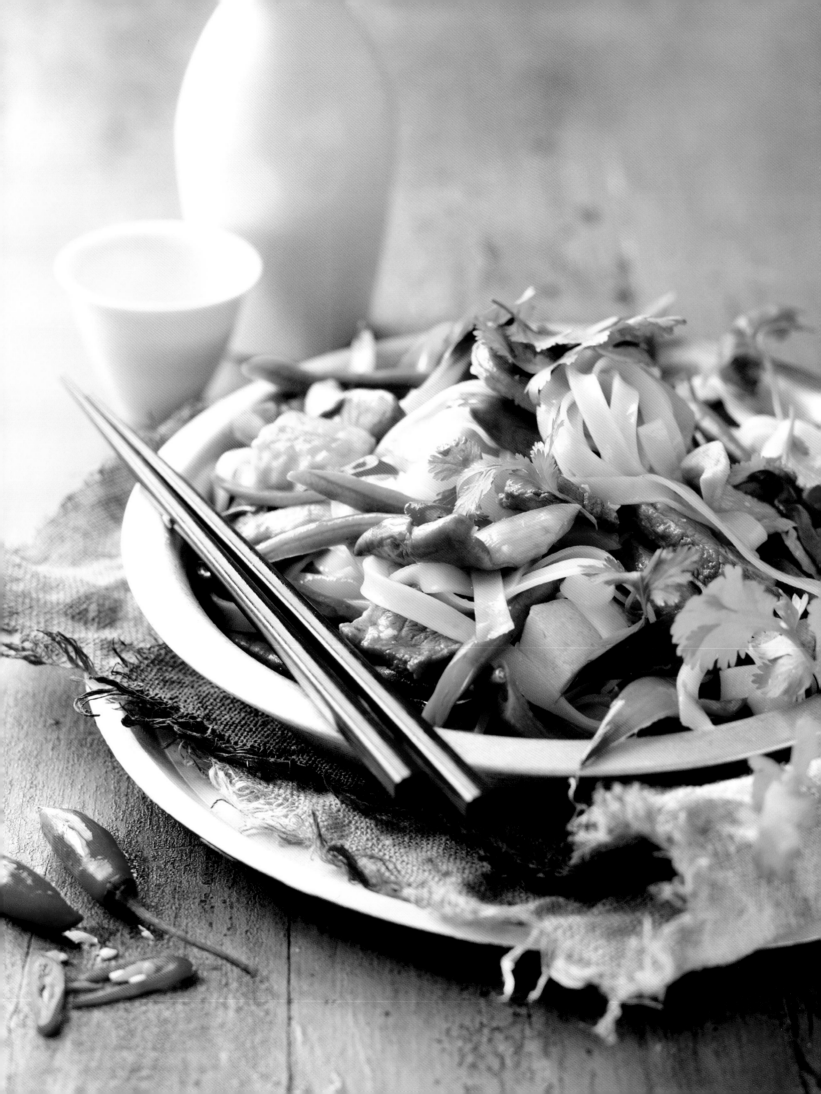

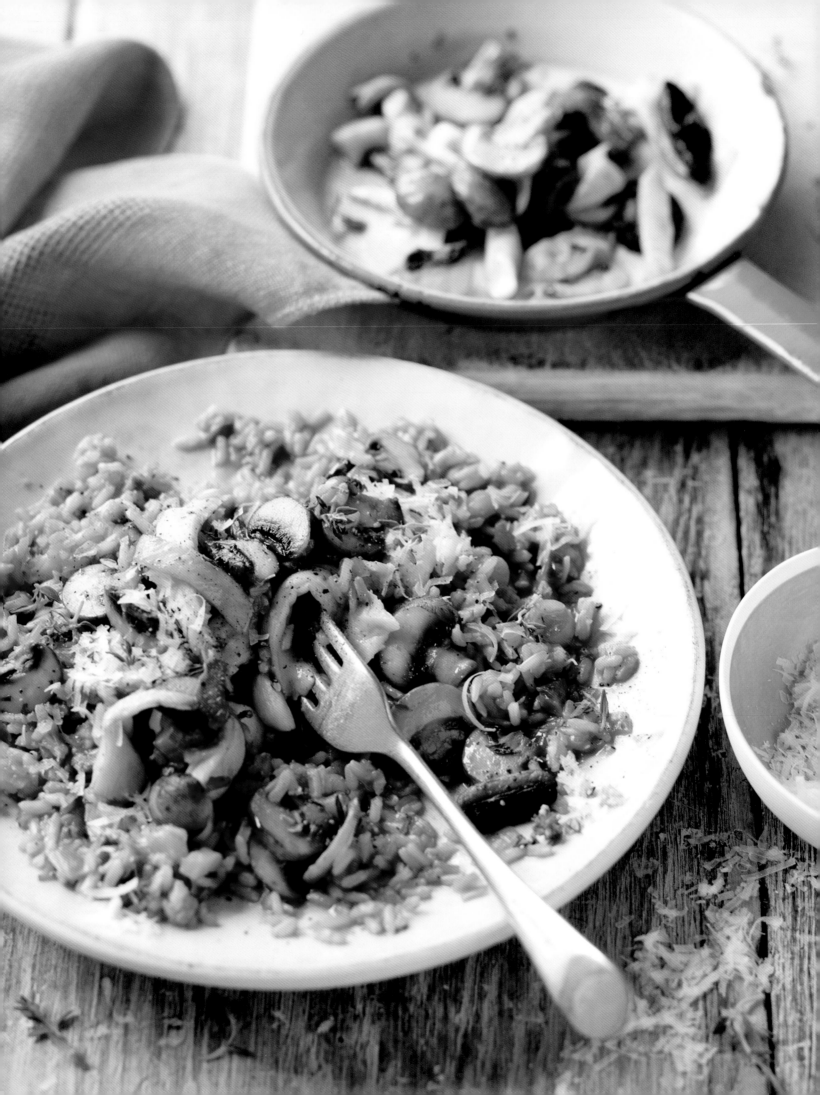

mushroom brown rice risotto

PREP + COOK TIME 1½ HOURS ◆ **SERVES** 2

20g (½ ounce) dried porcini or mixed mushrooms

1.625 litres (6½ cups) water

½ cup (125ml) water, extra

1 small leek (200g), sliced thinly

1 clove garlic, crushed

⅔ cup (130g) doongara low-GI brown rice

2 tablespoons finely grated pecorino cheese

2 teaspoons rice bran oil

75g (2 ounces) oyster mushrooms, sliced thinly

75g (2 ounces) swiss brown mushrooms, sliced thinly

½ teaspoon finely chopped fresh thyme

1 teaspoon lemon juice

1 teaspoon fresh thyme leaves, extra

1 Combine dried mushrooms and the water in a medium saucepan over medium heat, bring to a simmer. Remove from heat; stand for 15 minutes. Drain broth into a clean saucepan; reserve broth. Finely chop 2 teaspoons mushrooms, discard the remaining mushrooms. Return broth to heat; simmer, covered, over low heat.

2 Combine the extra water, leek and garlic in a medium saucepan over medium heat; cook, stirring occasionally, for 10 minutes or until leek is tender, (add an extra 1 tablespoon of water at a time if the pan becomes dry).

3 Add rice and reserved mushrooms to the pan, stirring to combine. Add 1 cup hot broth mixture; cook, stirring occasionally, over low heat, until broth is absorbed. Continue adding broth mixture, in 1-cup batches, stirring until absorbed between additions. Total cooking time should be approximately 50 minutes or until rice is tender. Stir half the cheese into the risotto.

4 Heat oil in a medium non-stick frying pan over high heat. Add oyster and swiss brown mushrooms and chopped thyme; cook, stirring occasionally, for 5 minutes or until mushrooms are browned lightly. Stir in juice, season with black pepper. Remove from heat; cover to keep warm.

5 Serve risotto topped with mushrooms, thyme leaves and remaining cheese.

TIP You could also use a combination of button and enoki mushrooms in this risotto.

barbecued squid with lemon cracked wheat risotto

PREP + COOK TIME 45 MINUTES ◆ **SERVES** 2

200g (6½ ounces) squid hoods, halved

1 clove garlic, crushed

2 teaspoons chopped fresh oregano

1 teaspoon finely grated lemon rind

1 tablespoon olive oil

1 small brown onion (80g), chopped finely

2 cloves garlic, crushed, extra

2 teaspoons fresh lemon thyme leaves

½ cup (80g) coarse cracked wheat

2 cups (500ml) water

1 cup (120g) frozen peas

1 tablespoon lemon juice

2 teaspoons fresh oregano leaves, extra

1   Score the inside of the squid with a small sharp knife; cut into 4cm (1½-inch) strips. Combine in a bowl with garlic, chopped oregano, rind and 2 teaspoons of oil.

2   Heat remaining oil in a medium non-stick frying pan over medium heat; cook onion, extra garlic and thyme, stirring, for 5 minutes or until softened.

3   Add cracked wheat and the water; cook, stirring occasionally, for 15 minutes or until cracked wheat is tender. Add peas and juice, stir for 2 minutes or until heated through.

4   Meanwhile, cook squid on a heated grill plate (or grill or barbecue) for 2 minutes, turning halfway through cooking time, or until just cooked through.

5   Slice squid. Serve cracked wheat with squid; sprinkle with extra oregano.

TIPS You could also try this with thin strips of chicken or pork. Cracked wheat can be bought from health food stores.

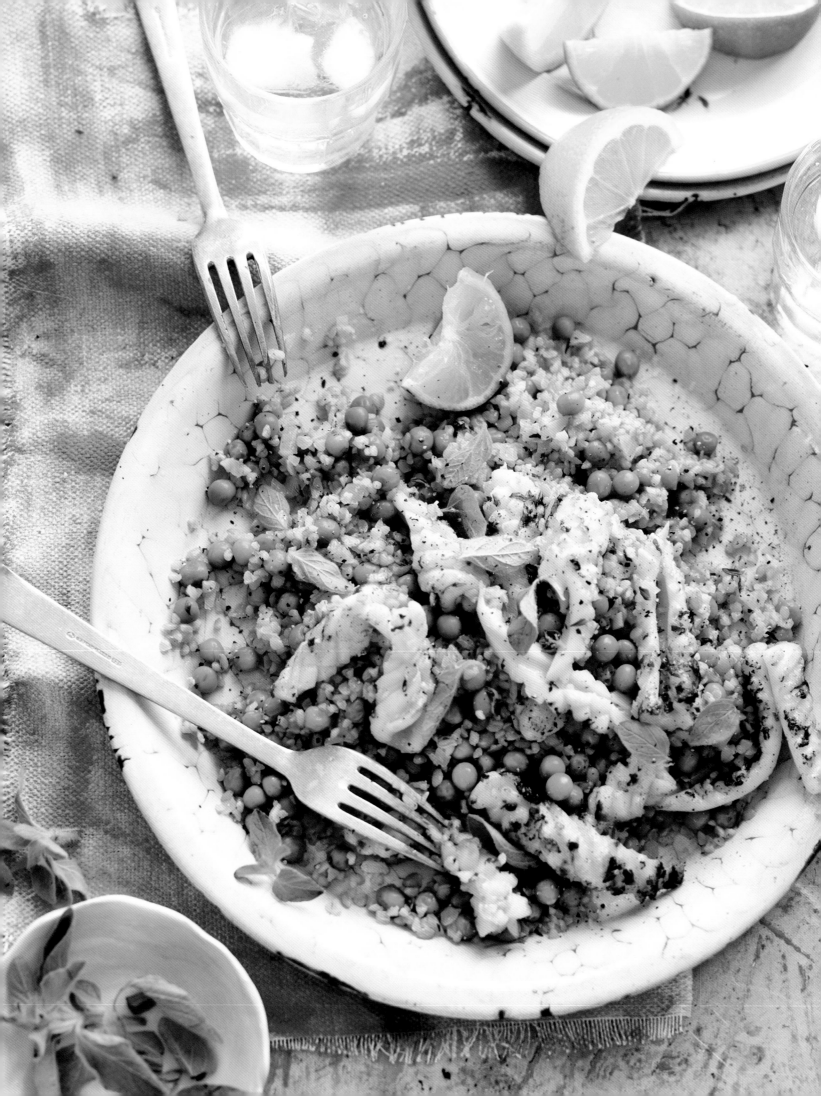

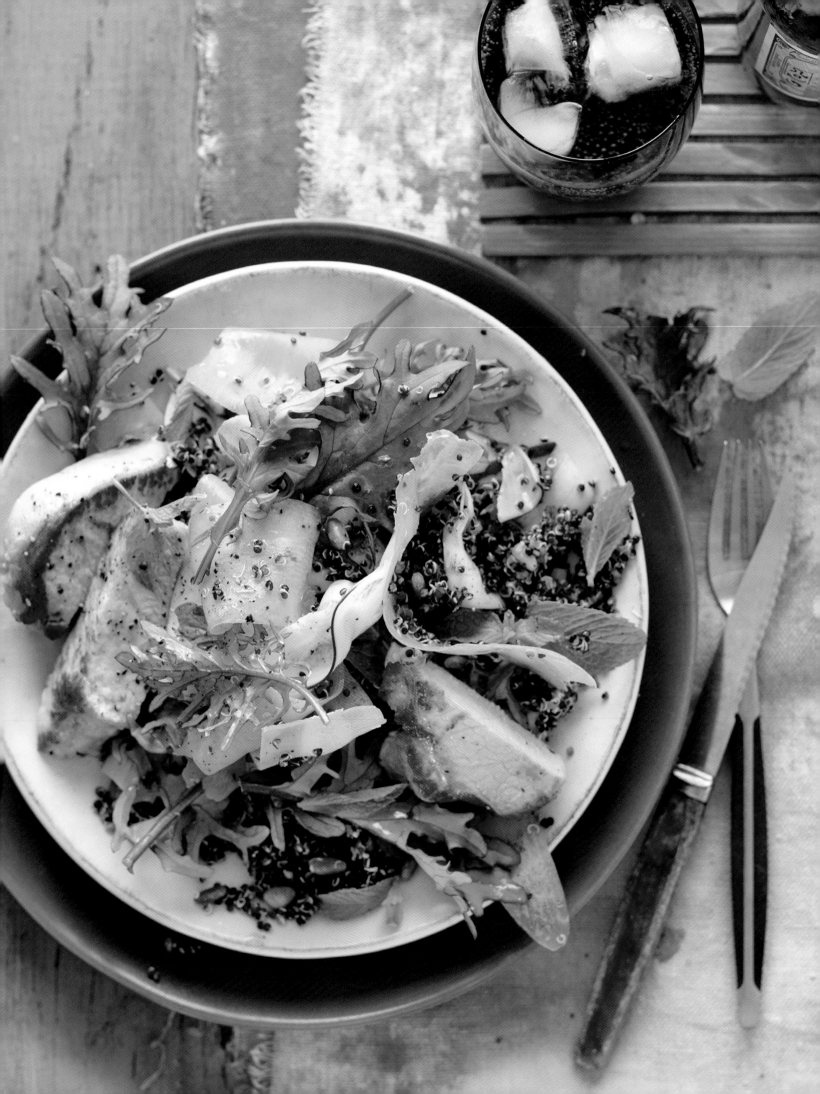

grilled pork with quinoa and kale salad

PREP + COOK TIME 30 MINUTES ◆ **SERVES** 2

⅓ cup (70g) black quinoa

1 small zucchini (90g), sliced into ribbons

1 medium carrot (120g), sliced into ribbons

1 small clove garlic, crushed

2 tablespoons lemon juice

1 tablespoon rice bran oil

2 x 125g (4 ounce) pork medallions

50g (1½ ounces) baby kale

1 tablespoon fresh mint leaves

2 teaspoons pine nuts, toasted

½ lemon (70g), cut into wedges

1 Rinse and drain quinoa well. Cook quinoa in a small saucepan of boiling water for 10 minutes or until tender; drain. Refresh under cold water; drain.

2 Meanwhile, place zucchini, carrot, garlic, juice and half the oil in a medium bowl; toss gently to combine.

3 Heat remaining oil in a small frying pan over high heat; cook pork for 3 minutes each side or until browned both sides and just cooked through.

4 Add quinoa, kale, mint and nuts to zucchini mixture; toss gently to combine.

5 Serve pork with salad and lemon wedges.

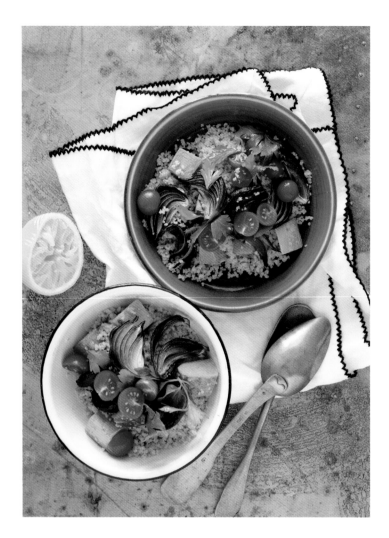

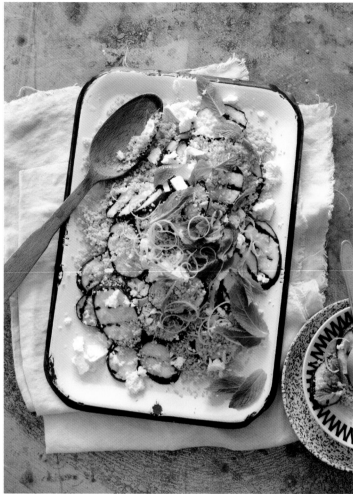

pumpkin tabbouleh

PREP + COOK TIME 35 MINUTES ◆ SERVES 2

Preheat oven to 220°C/425°F. Line oven tray with baking paper. Combine 200g (6½ ounces) chopped pumpkin and half a thickly sliced small red onion on tray; drizzle with 1 teaspoon olive oil. Bake for 20 minutes or until tender. Cool; transfer to a large bowl. Meanwhile, bring 1 cup water to the boil in a small saucepan. Add ⅓ cup cracked wheat; reduce heat, simmer, covered, for 15 minutes or until tender. Remove from heat; stand 10 minutes. Transfer to the bowl with vegetables. Combine ½ cup fresh flat-leaf parsley and 180g (5½ ounces) halved cherry tomatoes with pumpkin mixture. Combine 2 tablespoons lemon juice and 1 crushed garlic clove, drizzle over tabbouleh; toss gently to combine.

zucchini and mint couscous salad

PREP + COOK TIME 20 MINUTES ◆ SERVES 2

Combine ½ cup wholegrain couscous and ½ cup boiling water in a medium bowl; cover, stand for 5 minutes, fluff with a fork occasionally. Thickly slice 2 small zucchini; cook on a heated oiled grill plate (or grill or barbecue) for 2 minutes each side or until tender and browned. Combine zucchini, couscous, ½ cup fresh mint leaves, ¼ cup crumbled reduced-fat fetta, 1 tablespoon olive oil and 2 teaspoons each finely grated lemon rind and lemon juice.

TIP This is great as a side dish with grilled meats or fish.

NUTRITIONAL COUNT PER SERVING

- 5.5g total fat
- 0.8g saturated fat
- 877kJ (210 cal)
- 28.4g carbohydrate
- 6.3g protein
- 9.3g fibre
- 33mg sodium
- medium GI

NUTRITIONAL COUNT PER SERVING

- 13.4g total fat
- 3.7g saturated fat
- 1418kJ (339 cal)
- 38.4g carbohydrate
- 13.4g protein
- 5g fibre
- 285mg sodium
- medium GI

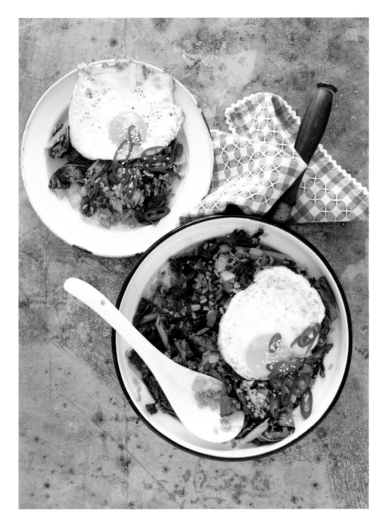
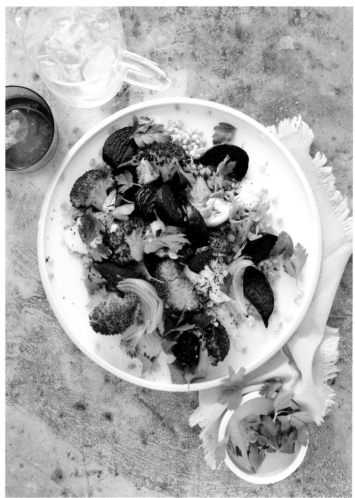

pearl barley salad

PREP + COOK TIME 50 MINUTES ◆ SERVES 2

Preheat oven to 220°C/425°F. Peel and cut 1 large beetroot (beet) and 1 medium brown onion into wedges; place on a large oven tray; drizzle with 2 teaspoons olive oil. Roast for 20 minutes. Add 200g (6½ ounces) broccoli florets; roast a further 15 minutes or until golden and tender. Meanwhile, cook ½ cup pearl barley in a medium saucepan of boiling water for 40 minutes or until tender; drain well. Combine 1 tablespoon each of tahini, warm water and lemon juice in a small bowl. Toss roasted vegetables and ½ cup fresh flat-leaf parsley through warm barley. Drizzle with tahini dressing to serve.

TIP You could use basmati or doongara as an alternative to brown rice. You will need ½ cup (100g) uncooked brown rice for this recipe.

NUTRITIONAL COUNT PER SERVING

- 12.3g total fat
- 14.7g protein
- 1.6g saturated fat
- 16.9g fibre
- 1576kJ (377 cal)
- 113mg sodium
- 43g carbohydrate
- low GI

brown rice and kale stir-fry

PREP + COOK TIME 15 MINUTES ◆ SERVES 2

Coarsely chop 1 medium brown onion. Coarsely chop the stalk and leaves of 100g (3 ounces) kale. Lightly spray a large non-stick frying pan with oil; cook onion and kale stalks, over medium heat, for 3 minutes. Stir in leaves, 1 cup cooked brown rice, 1 teaspoon grated fresh ginger and 2 teaspoons salt-reduced soy sauce; cook until hot. Transfer to a large bowl; cover to keep warm. Wipe pan clean. Lightly spray with cooking oil; cook 2 eggs, over low heat, until cooked. Serve rice topped with eggs. Sprinkle with ½ sliced long red chilli and 2 teaspoons toasted sesame seeds.

TIPS You could also use fresh mint or coriander. The salad tastes just as good at room temperature, so any leftovers will make a great packed lunch.

NUTRITIONAL COUNT PER SERVING

- 10.9g total fat
- 12.8g protein
- 2.4g saturated fat
- 5g fibre
- 1226kJ (293 cal)
- 258mg sodium
- 33.3g carbohydrate
- high GI

4 WAYS WITH RICE

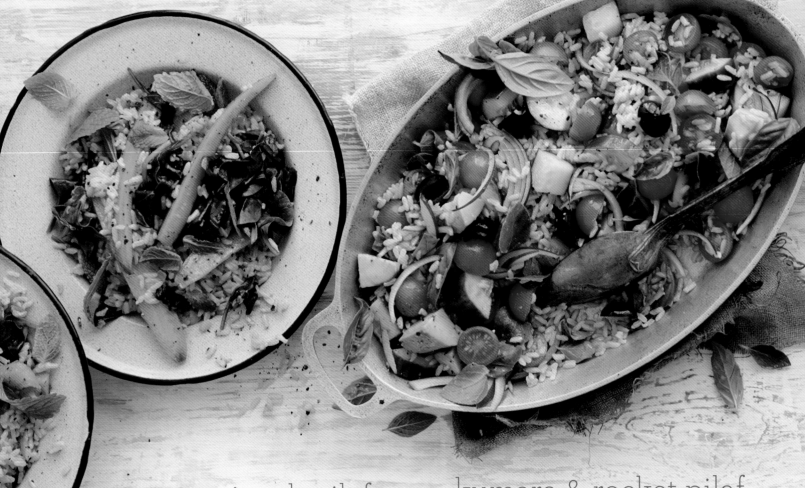

carrot & spinach pilaf

PREP + COOK TIME 45 MINUTES ◆ **SERVES** 2

Heat 2 teaspoons of olive oil in a medium saucepan over medium-high heat; cook 6 halved baby carrots for 5 minutes or until browned. Remove from pan. Cook half a finely chopped small brown onion in same pan, stirring, for 3 minutes or until softened. Stir in ¾ cup low-GI doongara brown rice and 1½ cups water; bring to the boil. Reduce heat; simmer, covered, for 25 minutes or until the rice is tender, returning carrots to the pan for the last 10 minutes of cooking time. Stir in 40g (1½ ounces) baby spinach leaves and 1 tablespoon small fresh mint leaves.

NUTRITIONAL COUNT PER SERVING

- 6.9g total fat
- 1.2g saturated fat
- 1395kJ (333 cal)
- 57.3g carbohydrate
- 7.3g protein
- 5.4g fibre
- 29mg sodium
- low GI

kumara & rocket pilaf

PREP + COOK TIME 45 MINUTES ◆ **SERVES** 2

Heat 2 teaspoons of olive oil in a medium saucepan over a medium-high heat; cook 150g (4½ ounces) coarsely chopped kumara (orange sweet potato) and half a finely chopped small brown onion, stirring, for 5 minutes or until onion softens. Stir in ⅔ cup low-GI doongara brown rice and 1⅓ cups water; bring to the boil. Reduce heat to low, cover; simmer, for 25 minutes or until the rice is tender. Stir in 30g (1 ounce) baby rocket leaves (arugula) and 1 tablespoon toasted pepitas.

NUTRITIONAL COUNT PER SERVING

- 9.4g total fat
- 1.5g saturated fat
- 1615kJ (386 cal)
- 63g carbohydrate
- 9.3g protein
- 5.3g fibre
- 18mg sodium
- low GI

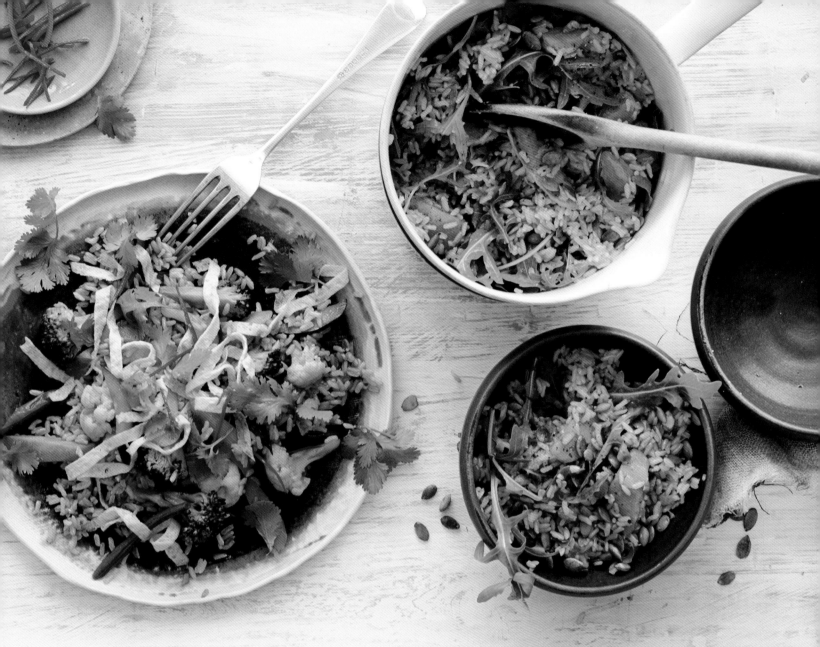

brown fried rice

PREP + COOK TIME 45 MINUTES ◆ **SERVES** 2

Cook ⅔ cup low-GI doongara brown rice in a large pan of boiling water for 25 minutes or until tender; drain. Heat 2 teaspoons of peanut oil in a large wok over a medium-high heat; swirl 1 lightly beaten egg to coat base of pan, cook for 1 minute or until just set. Transfer to a plate; slice egg thinly. Heat 2 teaspoons peanut oil in wok over medium-high heat; stir-fry 2 cups fresh or frozen stir-fry vegetable mix and 2 tablespoons water for 5 minutes or until just tender. Add rice to wok with 2 teaspoons kecap manis; stir to combine. Stir in egg and ⅓ cup fresh coriander leaves (cilantro). Serve fried rice topped with sliced fresh long red chilli, if you like.

NUTRITIONAL COUNT PER SERVING

- 10.9g total fat
- 2.7g saturated fat
- 1744kJ (417 cal)
- 59.6g carbohydrate
- 12.9g protein
- 13.8g fibre
- 447mg sodium
- low GI

greek brown rice salad

PREP + COOK TIME 50 MINUTES ◆ **SERVES** 2

Place ¾ cup low-GI long grain brown rice and 1½ cups water in a small saucepan; bring to the boil, then simmer, covered, for 25 minutes or until tender. Remove from heat; stand, covered, for 5 minutes. Add 6 pitted halved black olives, 1 chopped lebanese cucumber, ½ chopped small avocado, 1 cup halved cherry tomatoes, ½ thinly sliced small red onion and 2 tablespoons each fresh oregano and basil leaves. Combine 2 tablespoons red wine vinegar, 3 teaspoons rice bran oil and 1 crushed garlic clove; pour dressing over salad, toss to combine.

NUTRITIONAL COUNT PER SERVING

- 19.3g total fat
- 3.5g saturated fat
- 1942kJ (464 cal)
- 59.2g carbohydrate
- 8.5g protein
- 7.2g fibre
- 211mg sodium
- low GI

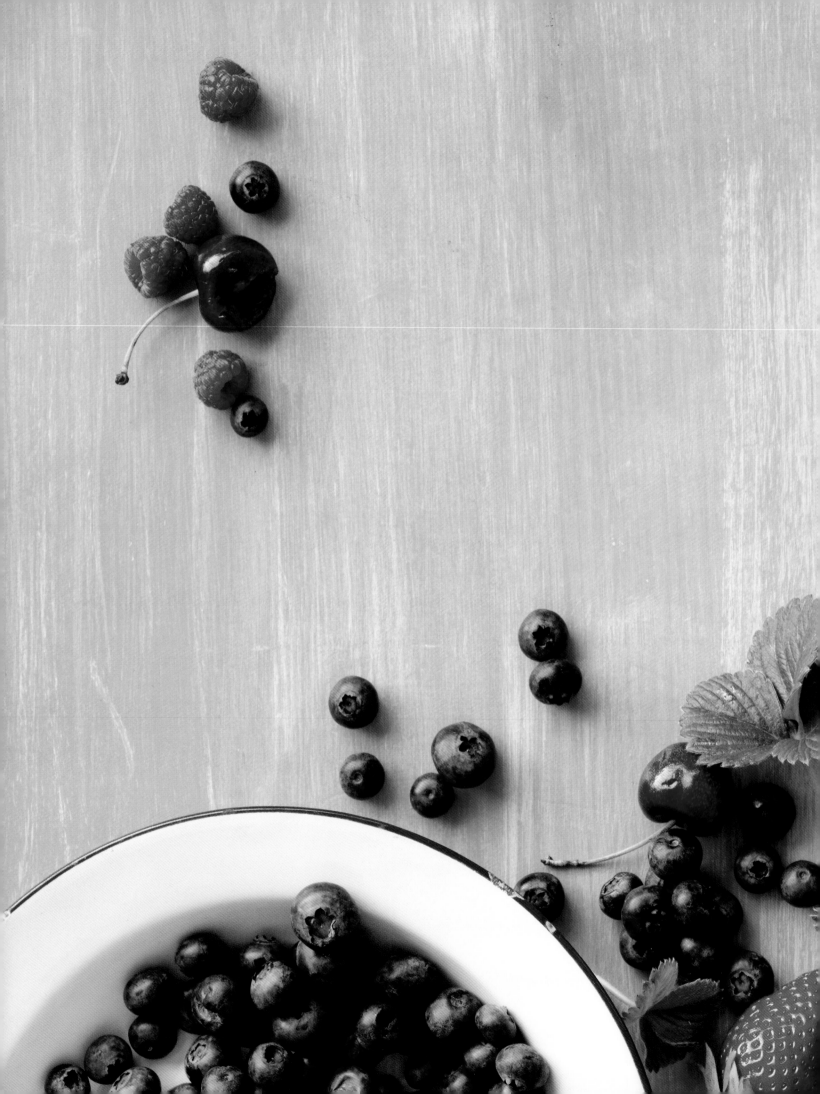

DESSERT

You can have your dessert and eat it too. Healthy eating doesn't mean you miss out on all the sweet stuff.

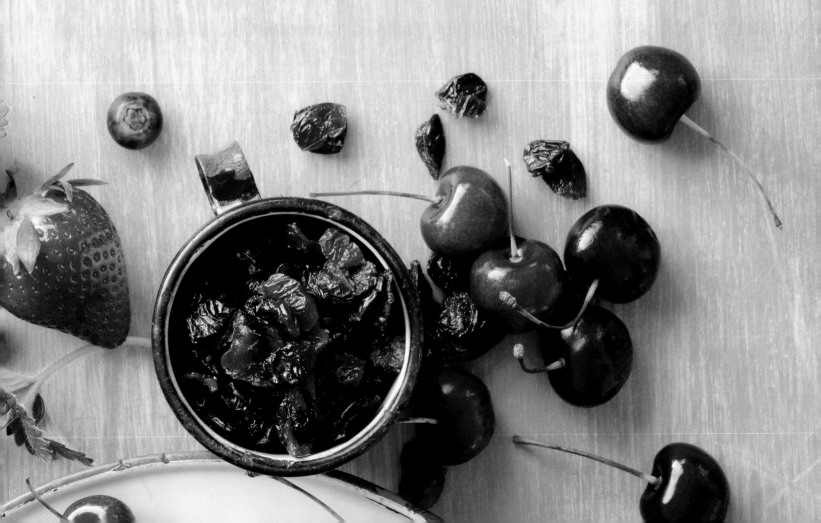

NUTRITIONAL COUNT PER SERVING

- 9.1g total fat
- 1.1g saturated fat
- 1067kJ (255 cal)
- 33g carbohydrate
- 12.2g protein
- 2.9g fibre
- 133mg sodium
- low GI

spelt crêpes with rhubarb in rose syrup

PREP + COOK TIME 40 MINUTES (+ REFRIGERATION) ◆ **SERVES** 2

⅓ cup (50g) white spelt flour

⅓ cup (80ml) skim milk

1 tablespoon grape-seed oil

1 egg white

1 teaspoon low-GI cane sugar

175g (5½ ounces) trimmed rhubarb, cut into 3cm (1¼-inch) lengths

1 tablespoon rose syrup

cooking-oil spray

½ cup (140g) low-fat plain yoghurt

1 Preheat grill (broiler). Line oven tray with baking paper.

2 Place flour, milk, oil, egg white and half the sugar in a medium bowl; whisk until smooth. Cover, refrigerate 30 minutes.

3 Meanwhile, place rhubarb on tray; sprinkle with remaining sugar and drizzle with syrup. Grill for 5 minutes or until rhubarb is tender.

4 Spray a heavy-based small non-stick frying pan with oil. Heat over medium-high heat; pour a sixth of the batter into pan. Cook until browned underneath. Turn crêpe, brown the other side. Repeat with remaining batter to make a total of 6 crêpes.

5 Serve crêpes with rhubarb and yoghurt.

TIP Rose syrup can be found in the international food aisle of major supermarkets or in specialty Middle-Eastern supermarkets. Substitute the rose syrup with half the amount of rose water, if you like.

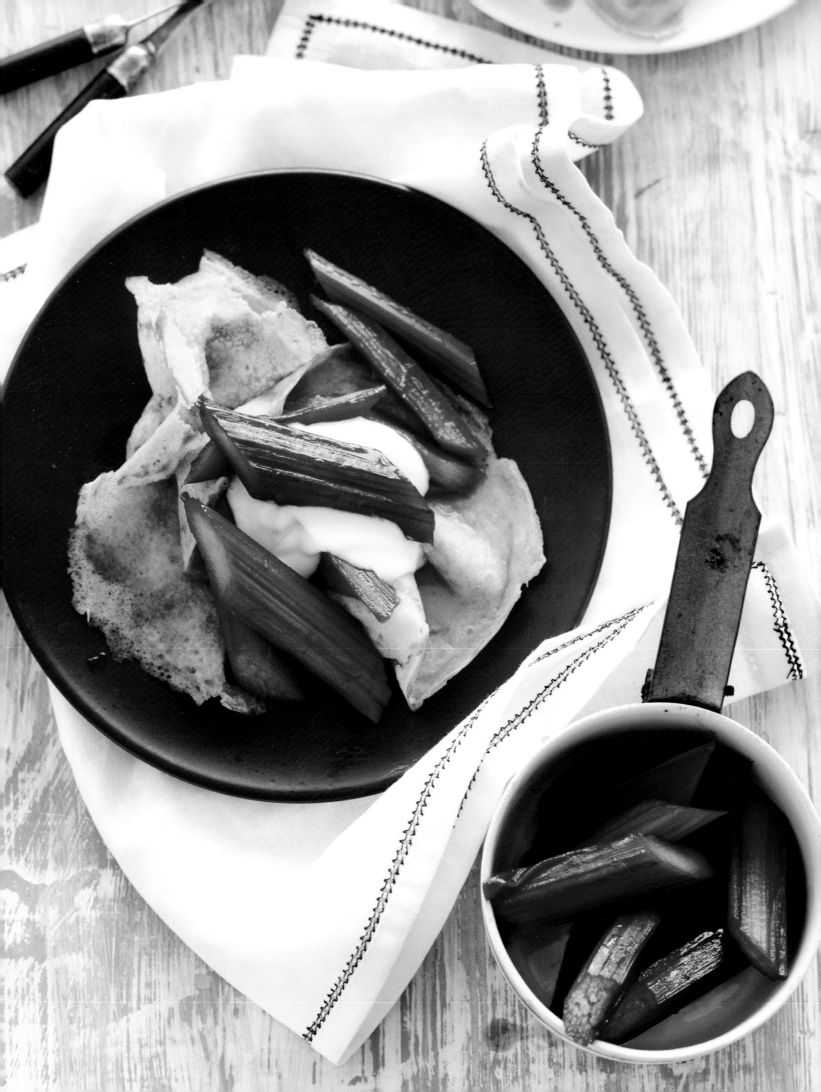

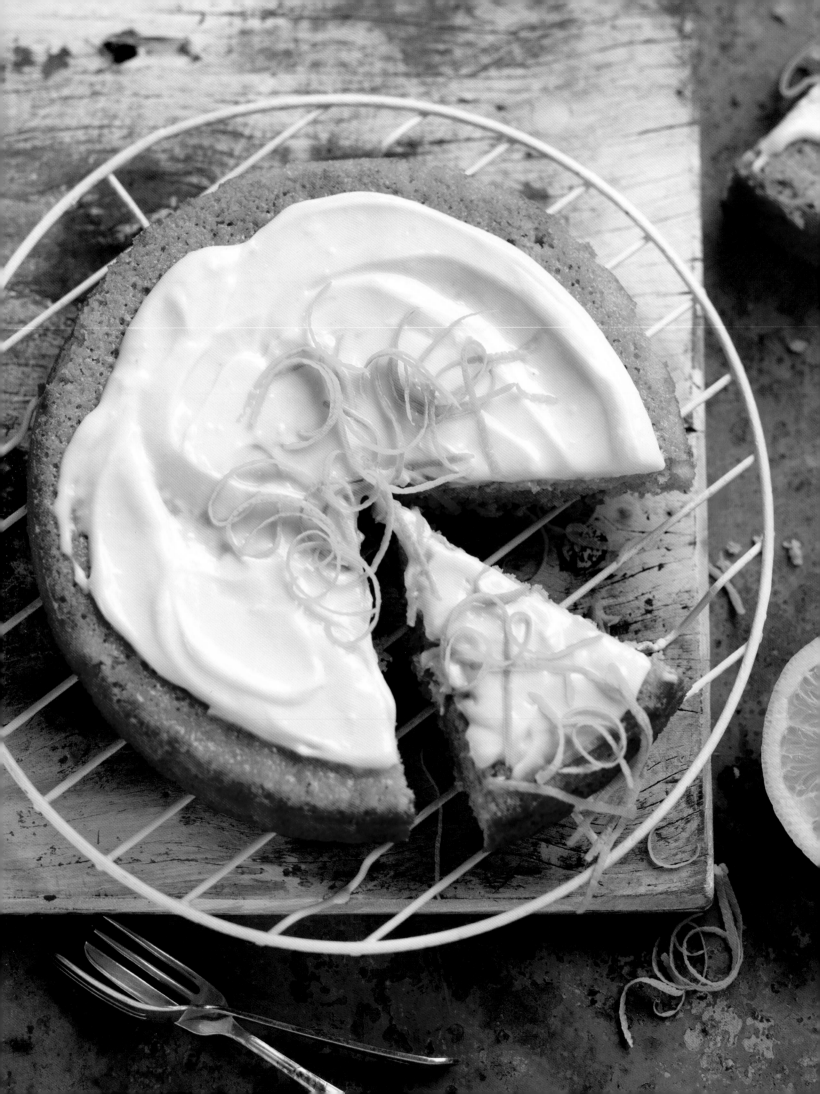

orange yoghurt cake

PREP + COOK TIME 55 MINUTES ◆ SERVES 12

2 eggs

¾ cup (165g) firmly packed brown sugar

2 teaspoons finely grated orange rind

¾ cup (90g) ground almonds

⅓ cup (50g) wholemeal self-raising flour

⅓ cup (95g) low-fat plain yoghurt

ORANGE CREAM CHEESE ICING

60g (2 ounces) light cream cheese, softened

2 tablespoons icing (confectioners') sugar

1 tablespoon orange juice

1　Preheat oven to 160°C/325°F. Grease a closed 20cm/8-inch (base measurement) round springform pan; line base and side with baking paper.

2　Beat eggs, sugar and rind in a small bowl with an electric mixer until light and fluffy. Stir in ground almonds, flour and yoghurt.

3　Spoon the mixture into pan; bake for about 45 minutes. Stand in pan for 5 minutes before turning, top-side up, onto a wire rack to cool.

4　Meanwhile, make orange cream cheese icing.

5　Spread cake with icing; top with thinly sliced orange rind, if you like.

ORANGE CREAM CHEESE ICING　Whisk ingredients in a small bowl until smooth.

TIPS Swap the orange for lemon for a citrus burst. The cake can be made ahead; store in an airtight container for up to 2 days or wrap and freeze for up to 2 months.

NUTRITIONAL COUNT PER SERVING

- 5g total fat
- 0.6g saturated fat
- 691kJ (165 cal)
- 27.9g carbohydrate
- 2.7g protein
- 1.5g fibre
- 58mg sodium
- medium GI

poached pears with espresso syrup

PREP + COOK TIME 55 MINUTES ◆ **SERVES** 2

2 small pears (360g)

1 vanilla bean, halved lengthways

1 tablespoon dark brown sugar

½ teaspoon instant coffee granules

HAZELNUT WAFERS

1 egg white

2 tablespoons caster (superfine) sugar

1 tablespoon ground hazelnut

1 tablespoon plain (all-purpose) flour

15g (½ ounce) low-fat salt-reduced margarine, melted

1 Make hazelnut wafers.

2 Cover peeled pears with water in a medium saucepan; bring to the boil. Reduce heat; simmer, uncovered, for 30 minutes or until pears are tender.

3 Drain pears, reserving 1 cup of cooking liquid.

4 Combine reserved liquid, vanilla bean and sugar in same pan; bring to the boil, stirring. Add coffee, reduce heat to medium; simmer, uncovered, for 10 minutes or until syrup thickens slightly.

5 Drizzle syrup over pears, serve with wafers.

HAZELNUT WAFERS Preheat oven to 200°C/400°F. Combine ingredients in a small bowl. Spread mixture onto a lined oven tray to make six 11cm (4½-inch) rounds. Bake for 8 minutes or until golden and crisp around the edges. Cool on a wire rack.

TIPS Watch the hazelnut wafers while baking, as they can easily burn if left in the oven too long. The wafers can be made a day ahead; store in an airtight container.

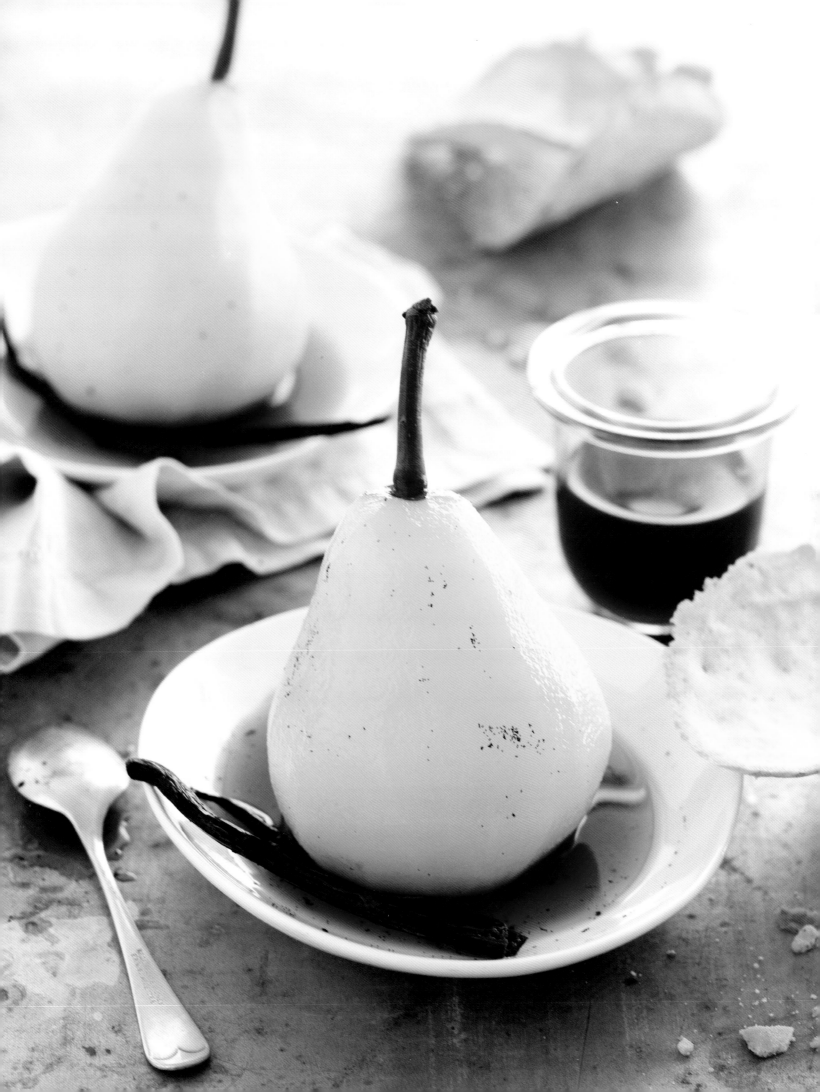

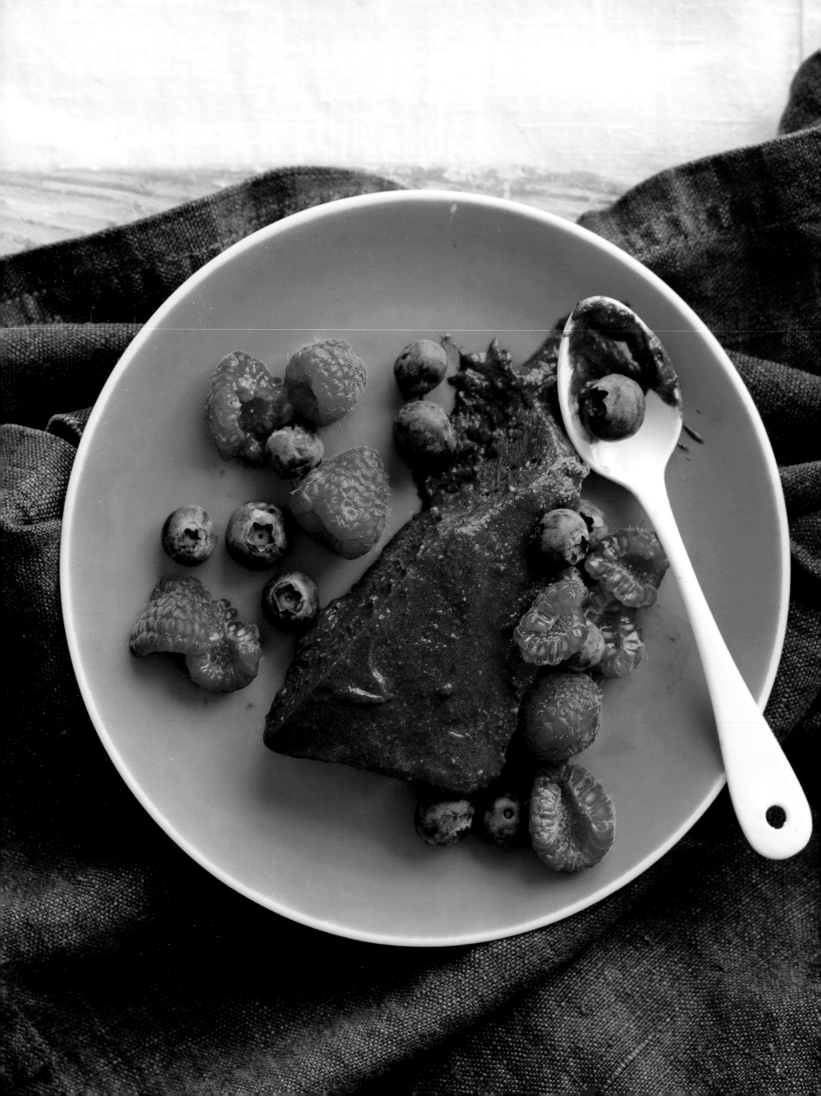

NUTRITIONAL COUNT PER SERVING

- 5.3g total fat
- 2.5g saturated fat
- 812kJ (194 cal)
- 27.3g carbohydrate
- 8.8g protein
- 2.9g fibre
- 122mg sodium;
- medium GI

chocolate semifreddo

PREP + COOK TIME 10 MINUTES (+ FREEZING) ◆ **SERVES** 2

1 tablespoon cocoa powder

¼ cup (40g) icing (confectioners') sugar

1 egg, separated

¼ cup (70g) low-fat ricotta

100g (3 ounces) fresh mixed berries

1 Lightly grease one ¾-cup (180ml) hole of a mini loaf pan. Line base and two long sides with baking paper, extending paper 2cm (¾-inch) above edges.
2 Whisk sifted cocoa and icing sugar, egg yolk and ricotta in a small bowl until smooth.
3 Beat egg white in a small bowl with an electric mixer until soft peaks form; fold through chocolate mixture, in two batches. Spoon into pan hole. Freeze for 4 hours or overnight.
4 Remove pan from freezer 10 minutes before serving. Cut in half and serve topped with berries.

NUTRITIONAL COUNT PER SERVING

- 5g total fat
- 2g saturated fat
- 732kJ (175 cal)
- 14.6g carbohydrate
- 12.8g protein
- 8.4g fibre
- 40mg sodium
- low GI

passionfruit mousse

PREP TIME 10 MINUTES (+ REFRIGERATION) ◆ **SERVES** 2

300g (9½ ounces) silken tofu

1 tablespoon light agave syrup

1 teaspoon vanilla extract

1 teaspoon finely grated lemon rind

¼ cup (60ml) fresh passionfruit pulp

1 tablespoon fresh mint leaves

1 tablespoon fresh passionfruit pulp, extra

1 tablespoon flaked coconut, toasted

1 Blend or process tofu, syrup, vanilla and rind until smooth. Stir through passionfruit.

2 Spoon mixture into two 1-cup (250ml) serving glasses. Refrigerate for 2 hours.

3 Serve mousse topped with mint, extra passionfruit and coconut.

TIP You will need about 3 passionfruit.

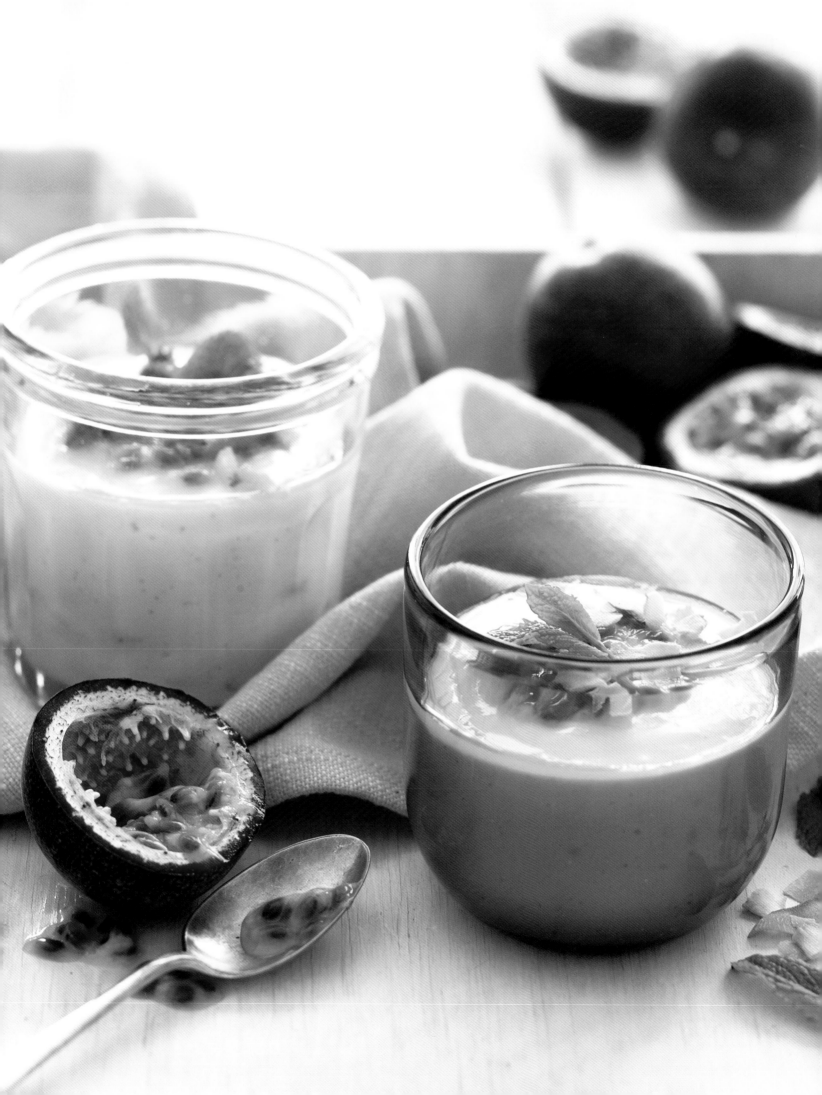

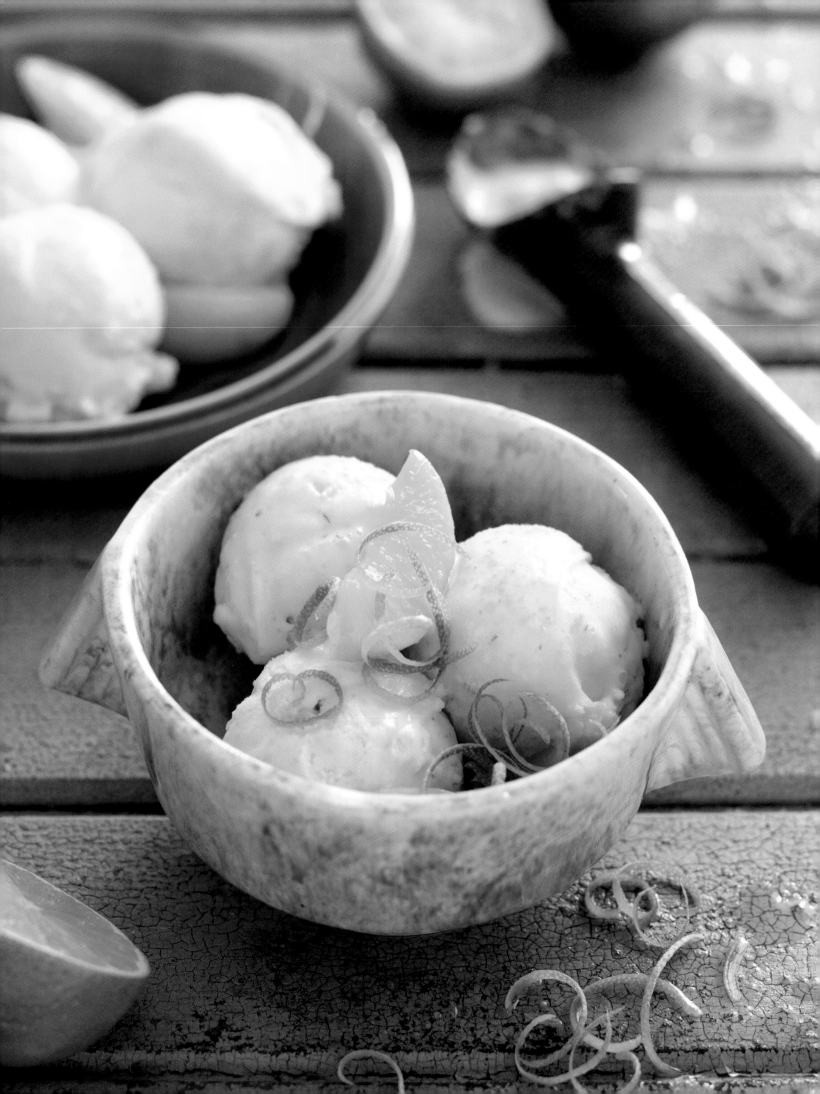

frozen peach lassi

PREP + COOK TIME 10 MINUTES (+ FREEZING) ◆ **SERVES** 4

2 cups (365g) drained canned peach slices in natural juice

2 tablespoons honey

½ cup (125ml) buttermilk

1 cup (280g) low-fat plain yoghurt

2 teaspoons finely grated lime rind

2 teaspoons lime juice

1 cup (180g) canned peach slices in natural juice, extra

1 teaspoon finely grated lime rind, extra

Lassi is a yoghurt-based drink from India.

1 Process or blend peaches until smooth.

2 Whisk peach puree with the honey, buttermilk, yoghurt, rind and juice in a large bowl.

3 Pour mixture into a 1-litre (4-cup) container. Cover tightly with foil; freeze for 3 hours or overnight.

4 Beat lassi in a large bowl with an electric mixer until smooth. Return to container, cover; freeze a further 3 hours or until firm. Alternatively, churn lassi in an ice-cream machine according to the manufacturer's instructions.

5 Serve lassi with extra peach slices and lime rind.

TIPS You will need a 1kg (2 pound) container of peach slices in natural juice for this recipe. You could also try this with other canned fruits such as plum or mango.

strawberry and orange mille feuille

PREP + COOK TIME 15 MINUTES (+ COOLING) ◆ SERVES 2

cooking-oil spray

1 sheet fillo pastry

⅓ cup (80g) low-fat ricotta

1 tablespoon icing (confectioners') sugar

½ teaspoon finely grated orange rind

3 teaspoons orange juice

325g (8 ounces) strawberries, sliced thinly

1 Preheat oven to 200°C/400°F. Lightly spray a baking tray with oil.

2 Lightly spray pastry with oil; fold in half. Cut pastry into six rectangles. Place on tray; bake for 5 minutes or until golden. Cool.

3 Meanwhile, combine ricotta, 3 teaspoons of the sifted icing sugar, rind and juice in a bowl.

4 Place a pastry rectangle on a serving plate; lightly spread a quarter of the ricotta mixture over pastry, top with a quarter of the strawberries. Repeat layer, finishing with a third pastry rectangle.

5 Repeat step 4 to make a second mille feuille; sprinkle mille feuilles with the remaining sifted icing sugar to serve.

TIPS To avoid the mille feuille slipping around the plate, place a dab of the ricotta mixture under the first pastry rectangle. It will hold the pastry in place. You need to assemble these mille feuilles just before serving or the pastry will go soggy. You can use any seasonal fruit such as raspberries and blueberries, thinly sliced stone fruit, or sliced seedless grapes or fresh figs.

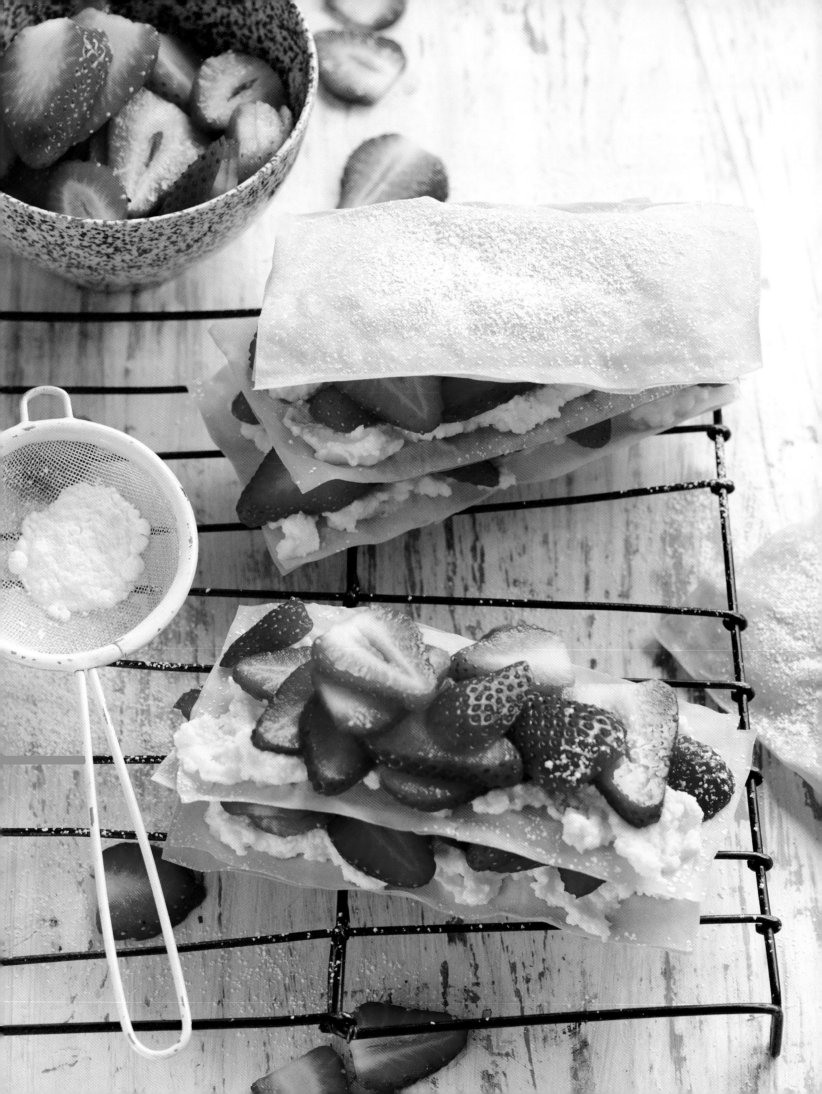

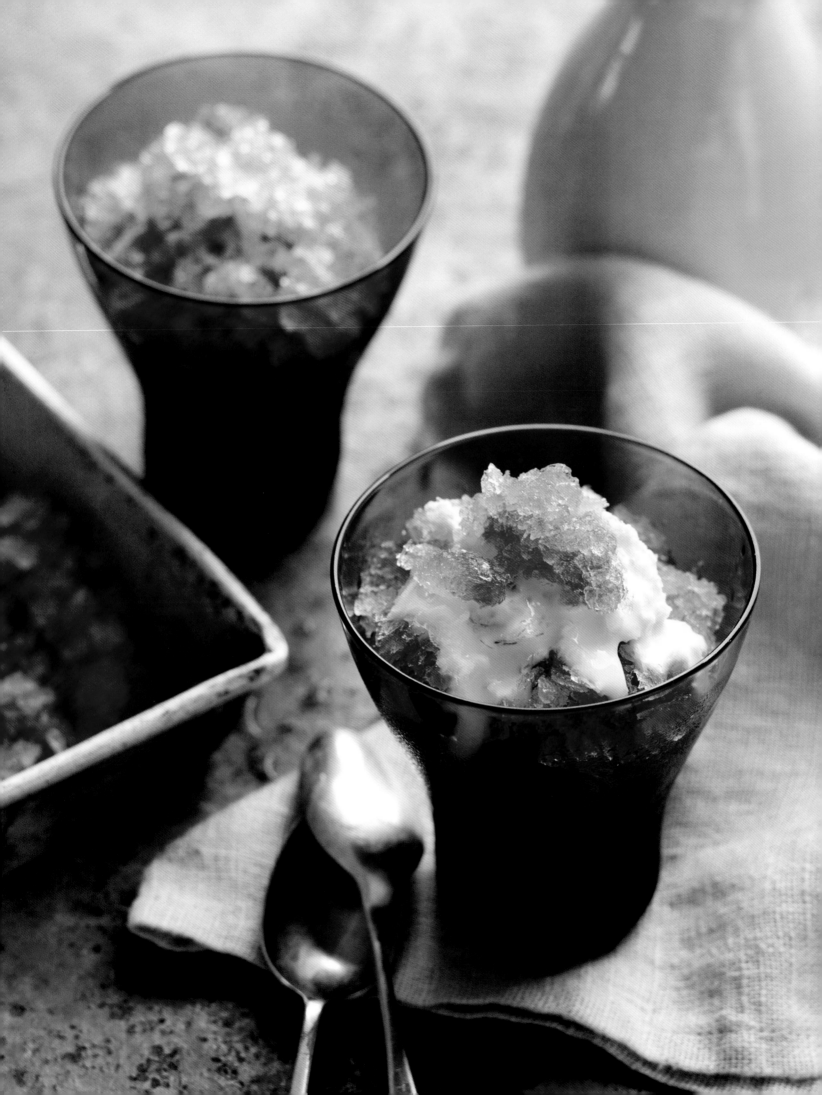

NUTRITIONAL COUNT PER SERVING

- 1.8g total fat
- 1.2g saturated fat
- 279kJ (67 cal)
- 12.9g carbohydrate
- 0.3g protein
- 2.9g fibre
- 3mg sodium
- low GI

coffee granita

PREP + COOK TIME 10 MINUTES (+ COOLING & FREEZING) ◆ SERVES 6

⅓ cup (75g) low-GI cane sugar

3 cups (750ml) water

¼ cup (60ml) strong espresso coffee

¼ cup (60ml) thickened (heavy) light cream

1 Combine sugar and the water in a small saucepan over low heat, stirring, until sugar is dissolved. Remove from heat, stir in coffee, cool to room temperature.

2 Pour coffee mixture into a shallow metal tray; cover, freeze for 6 hours, scraping with a fork every hour.

3 Scrape granita with a fork; spoon into glasses, drizzle each with 2 teaspoons of cream; serve granita immediately.

TIPS To make the strong espresso coffee, dissolve 3 teaspoons instant espresso coffee into 1/3 cup boiling water. This granita is a delicious alternative to regular coffee for brunch when entertaining friends in the warmer months. Use granita within 1 month of making.

NUTRITIONAL COUNT PER SERVING

- 4.4g total fat
- 1g saturated fat
- 607kJ (145 cal)
- 17.2g carbohydrate
- 2.1g protein
- 2.4g fibre
- 124mg sodium
- low GI

strawberry and pomegranate baked custard tarts

PREP + COOK TIME 20 MINUTES ◆ SERVES 2

1 sheet fillo pastry

cooking-oil spray

⅔ cup (160ml) low-fat milk

1 egg

2 teaspoons caster (superfine) sugar

½ teaspoon vanilla extract

6 small strawberries (75g), quartered lengthways

40g (1½ ounces) fresh pomegranate seeds

1 teaspoon pomegranate molasses

1 Preheat oven to 200°C/400°F. Oil two holes of a 12-hole (⅓-cup/180ml) muffin pan.

2 Cut pastry in half crossways. Lightly spray one of the pastry halves with oil, then fold in half; cut pastry into four. Firmly press pastry strips into pan hole overlapping each other to cover hole, spray lightly with oil to stick pastry strips together. Repeat with remaining pastry.

3 Bake cases for 5 minutes or until pastry is browned lightly.

4 Meanwhile, heat milk until hot. Whisk egg, sugar and extract in a small bowl; gradually whisk in hot milk. Pour custard into pastry cases. Bake for 15 minutes or until set. Stand tarts for 5 minutes before transferring to a wire rack to cool.

5 Combine strawberries, pomegranate seeds and molasses in a small bowl. Serve tarts topped with strawberry mixture.

TIPS The tarts can be made a day ahead; store in an airtight container in the fridge. Top with the strawberry mixture before serving.

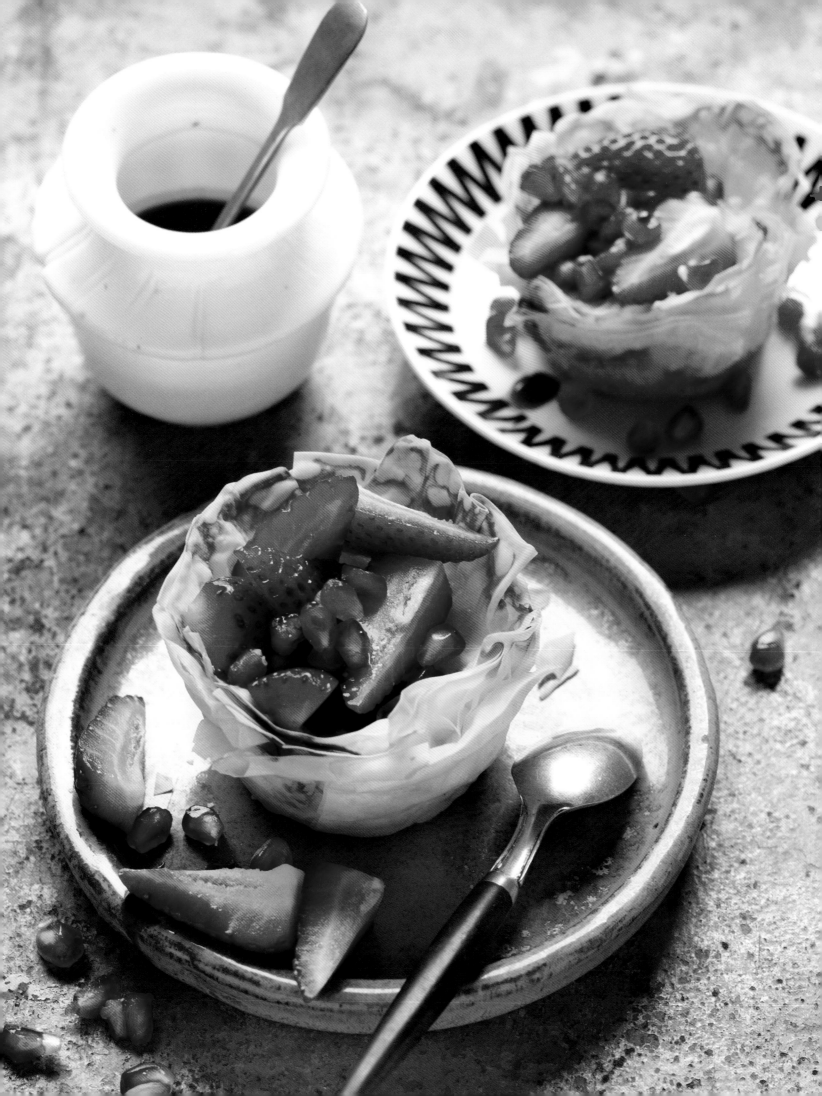

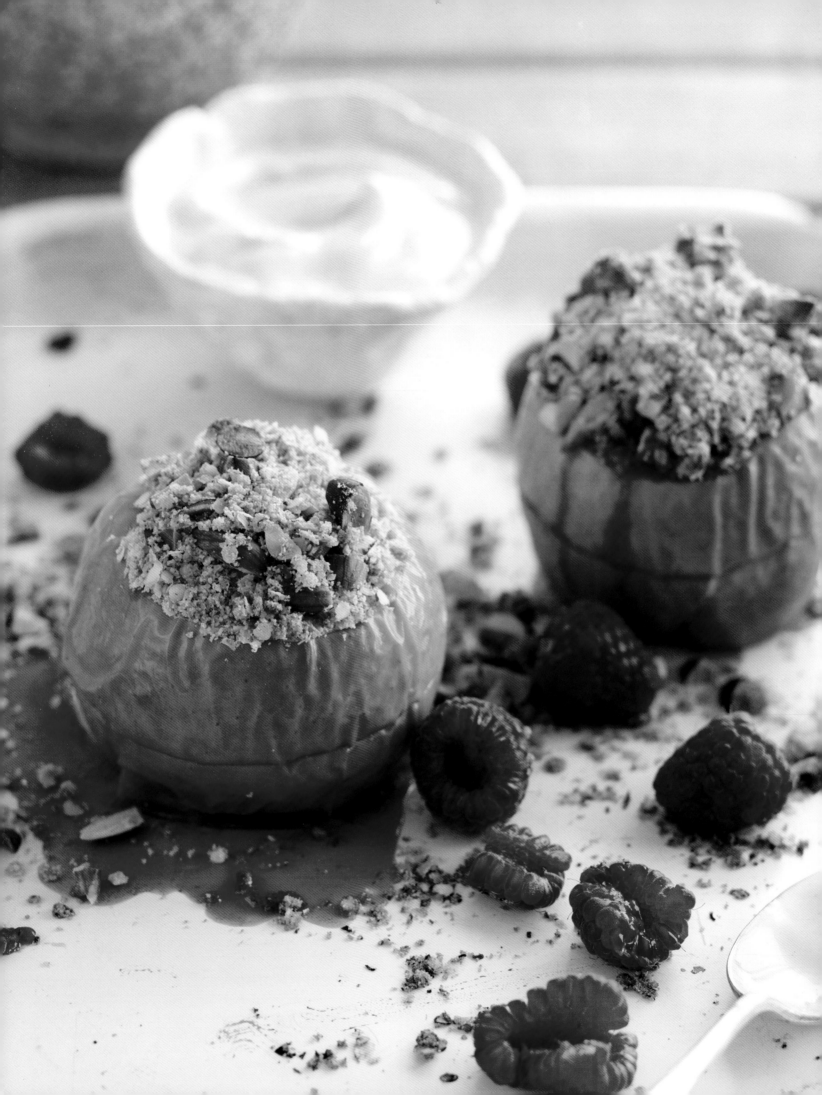

NUTRITIONAL COUNT PER SERVING

● 5.6g total fat ● 2.3g protein

● 1.5g saturated fat ● 5.7g fibre

● 770kJ (184 cal) ● 18mg sodium

● 28g carbohydrate ● low GI

baked apples and raspberries with quinoa almond crumble

PREP + COOK TIME 1 HOUR ◆ SERVES 2

2 medium pink lady apples (300g), unpeeled

50g (1½ ounces) fresh raspberries

1 teaspoon finely grated lemon rind

2 teaspoons low-GI cane sugar

CRUMBLE TOPPING

1 tablespoon quinoa flakes

2 teaspoons white spelt flour

1 tablespoon coarsely chopped roasted almonds

½ teaspoon low-GI cane sugar

1 teaspoon butter

pinch cinnamon

1 Preheat oven to 160°C/325°F. Grease and line a baking tray with baking paper.

2 Make crumble topping.

3 Core unpeeled apples about three-quarters of the way down from stem end, making the hole 4cm (1½ inches) in diameter. Use a small sharp knife to score around the centre of each apple. Make a small deep cut in the base of each apple.

4 Pack combined berries, rind and sugar firmly into apples; top with crumble topping. Place apples on tray. Bake, uncovered, for 45 minutes or until apples are just tender.

CRUMBLE TOPPING Place ingredients in a small bowl; using your fingers, rub the mixture together until well combined.

SERVING SUGGESTION Serve with low-fat ice-cream or yoghurt.

TIPS Use your favourite variety of apple; we used pink lady as they have a sweet flavour that marries well with the raspberries. If you don't have an apple corer, you can use a melon baller to remove the apple core.

tropical jelly with coconut yoghurt

PREP + COOK TIME 10 MINUTES (+ REFRIGERATION) ◆ **SERVES** 2

1 x 9g (½ ounce) sachet sugar-free mango and passionfruit jelly crystals

1 cup (250ml) boiling water

1 cup (250ml) cold water

1 small mango (300g), sliced

2 tablespoons coconut yoghurt

2 tablespoons fresh passionfruit pulp

1 tablespoon fresh mint leaves

1   Place jelly and the boiling water in a medium bowl. Stir to dissolve crystals. Add the cold water; stir to combine.

2   Divide mango between two 1½-cup (375ml) glasses; pour over jelly. Refrigerate for at least 4 hours or until set.

3   Top jellies with yoghurt, passionfruit and mint.

TIPS You can make these jellies the day ahead, just cover with plastic wrap and refrigerate. Top with yoghurt, passionfruit and mint just before serving.

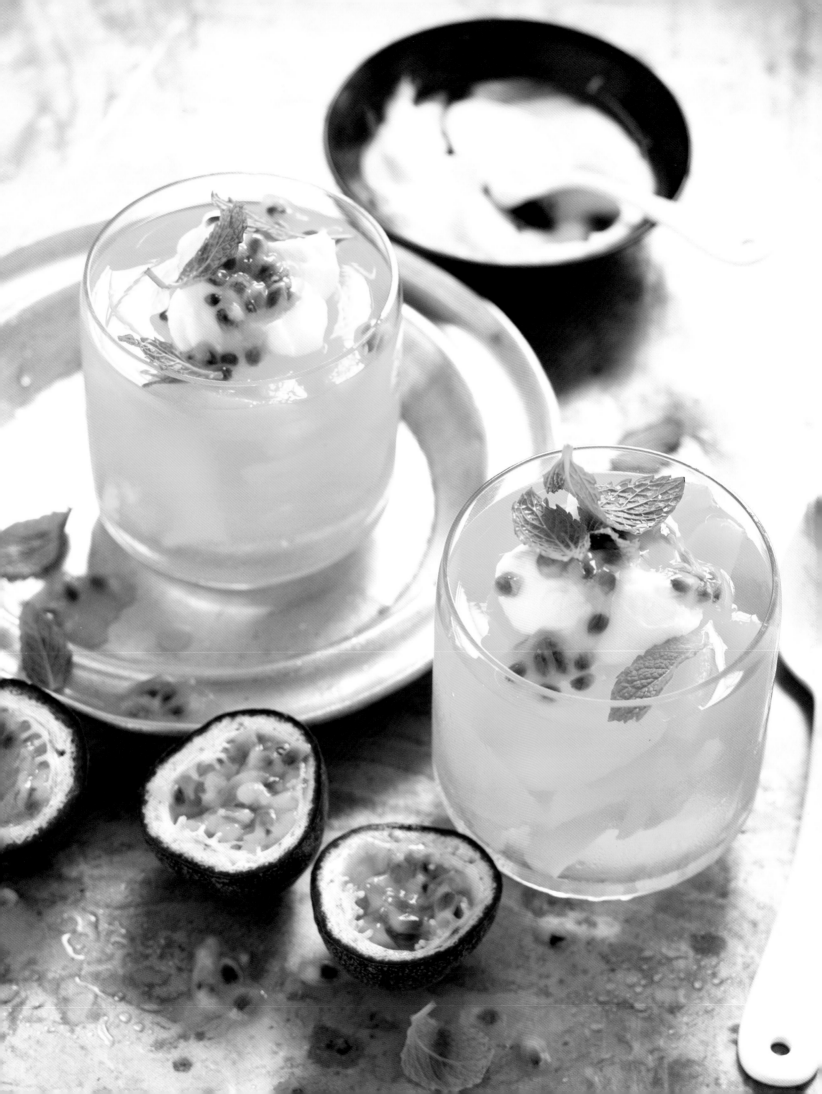

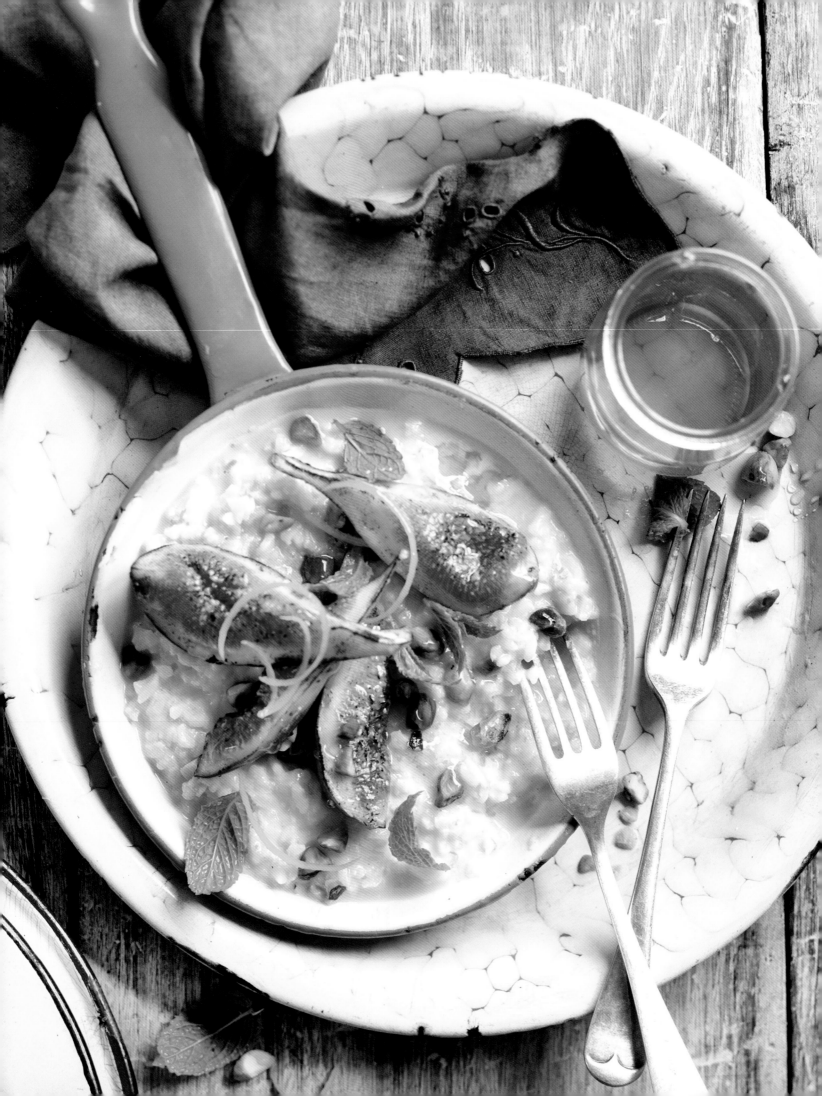

fig and orange blossom rice pudding

PREP + COOK TIME 55 MINUTES (+ STANDING) ◆ **SERVES** 2

¼ cup (50g) low-GI white rice

1 cup (250ml) skim milk

1 cinnamon stick

1 cardamom pod, bruised

1 small egg yolk

¼ teaspoon orange blossom water

2 teaspoons finely grated orange rind

1 fresh fig (60g), quartered

10 pistachios, chopped

2 teaspoons fresh mint leaves

2 teaspoons honey

1 Cook rice in a small saucepan of boiling water for 20 minutes or until soft. Drain well.

2 Meanwhile, heat milk, cinnamon and cardamom in a small non-stick saucepan over low heat. Bring just to a simmer, then remove from heat; cover and stand for 20 minutes to infuse.

3 Add rice to milk mixture; simmer over low heat for 10 minutes. Add egg yolk; stir over low heat for 30 seconds or until thickened slightly. Stir in orange blossom water and rind. Cool for 20 minutes or until mixture is warm. Discard cinnamon and cardamom.

4 Preheat grill (broiler) to high. Place figs on a foil-lined oven tray; grill for 3 minutes or until figs are browned and tender.

5 Spoon rice into 2 small serving glasses; top with figs and any juices, nuts and mint. Drizzle with honey.

roasted pears with cinnamon labne

PREP + COOK TIME I HOUR (+ REFRIGERATION) ◆ **SERVES** 2

½ cup (140g) low-fat greek yoghurt

1 herbal lemon tea bag

1 cup (250ml) boiling water

2 strips lemon rind

1 teaspoon honey

2 small firm pears (360gg), peeled, halved, cored

¼ teaspoon ground cinnamon

2 teaspoons chopped roasted hazelnuts

Start this recipe a day ahead.

1 Line a sieve or colander with muslin, place over a large bowl. Spoon yoghurt into muslin; cover with plastic wrap. Refrigerate overnight to drain; discard any liquid.

2 Preheat oven to 200°C/400°F.

3 Combine tea bag, the boiling water, rind and half the honey in a small bowl. Stand for 5 minutes. Drain; discard tea bag.

4 Place pears in a medium baking dish; pour over tea mixture. Transfer to oven; roast for 45 minutes, turning every 15 minutes, or until pears are tender.

5 Combine yoghurt, cinnamon and remaining honey in a small bowl.

6 Serve pears with yoghurt mixture; drizzle with any cooking liquid and sprinkle with nuts.

TIPS Use a melon baller to core the pears. You can use bought labne in this recipe if you are time poor, just be aware the nutritional count will change; make sure you check the label for the sodium and fat content.

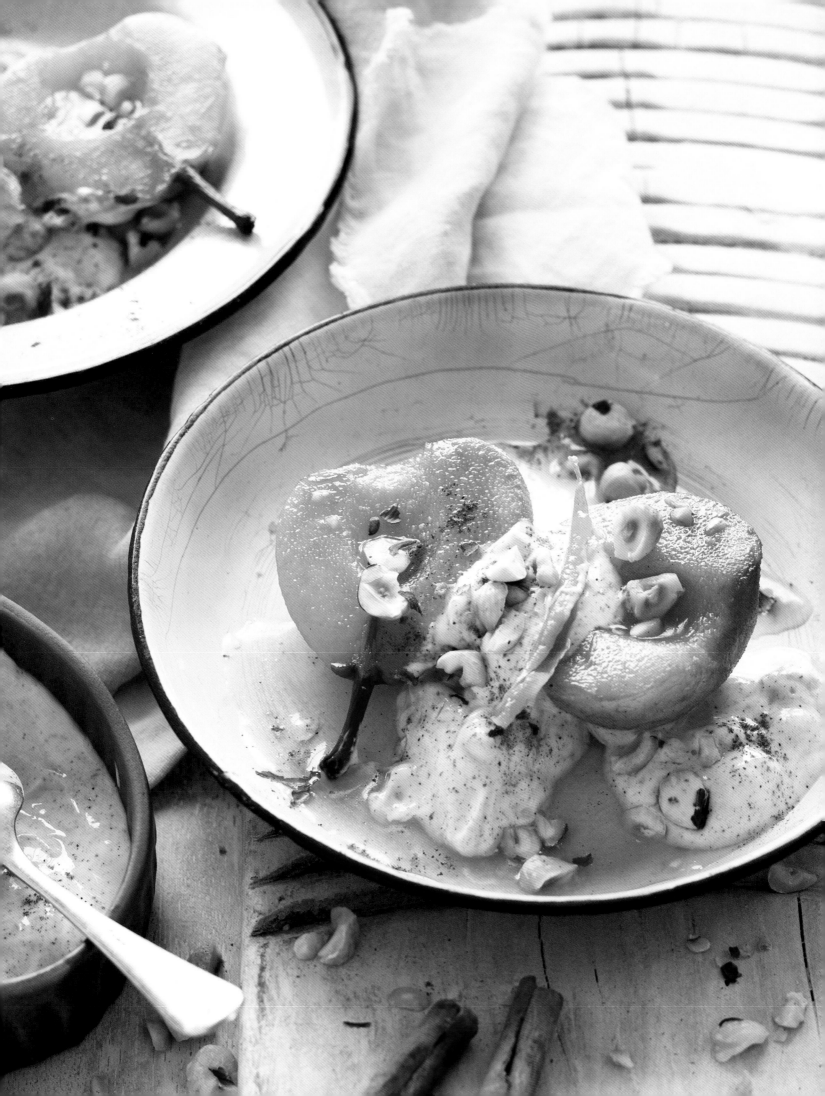

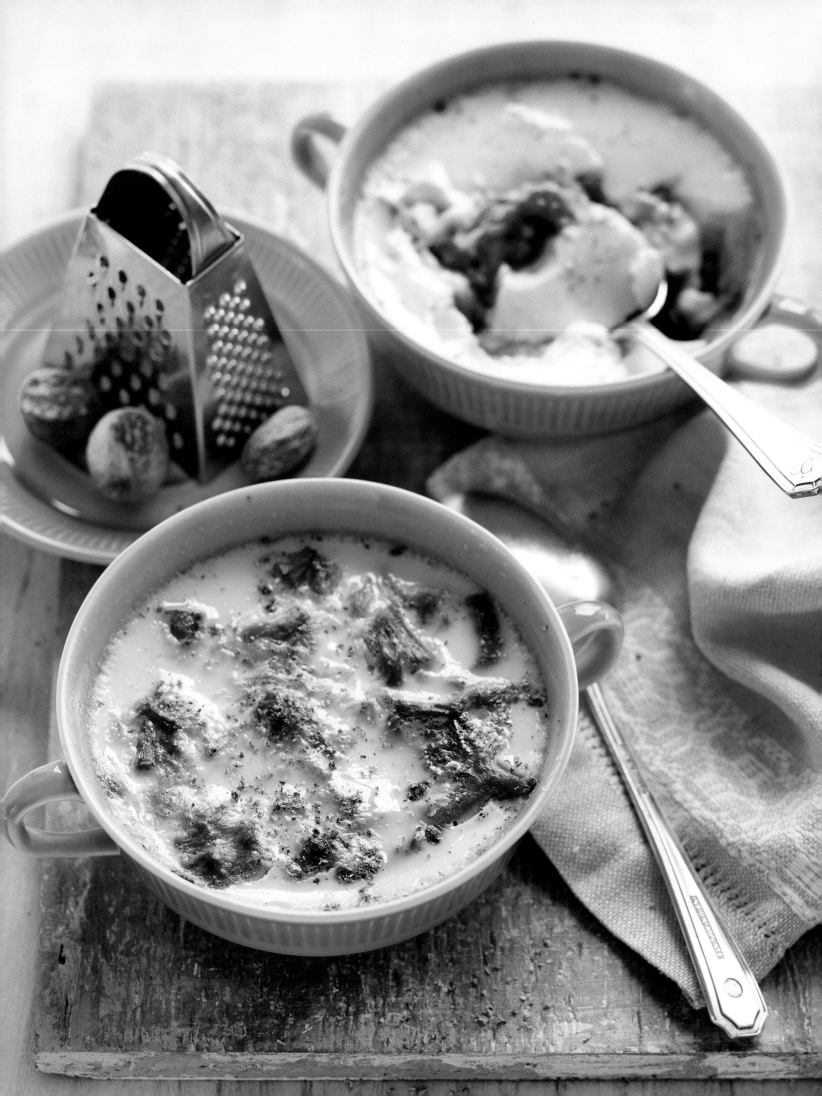

rhubarb and vanilla baked custard

PREP + COOK TIME 50 MINUTES ◆ **SERVES** 2

4 stems trimmed rhubarb (250g), chopped coarsely

2 tablespoons caster (superfine) sugar

1 vanilla bean, split lengthways

2 small eggs

1 cup (250ml) hot low-fat milk

pinch ground nutmeg

1 Preheat oven to 220°C/425°F. Grease and line a large baking tray. Grease two 1½-cup (375ml) ovenproof dishes.

2 Toss rhubarb with 2 teaspoons of the sugar on baking tray. Roast for 15 minutes or until rhubarb is tender. Mash rhubarb with a fork. Divide rhubarb between ovenproof dishes. Reduce oven temperature to 160°C/325°F.

3 Remove seeds from vanilla bean. Whisk eggs, vanilla seeds and remaining sugar in a medium bowl; whisk in hot milk. Gently pour custard mixture over rhubarb in dishes; sprinkle with nutmeg.

4 Place dishes in a medium baking dish; add enough boiling water to come halfway up side of dishes. Bake for 30 minutes or until custard is just set.

TIPS The rhubarb can be made up to 3 days in advance; store, covered, in the fridge. Place the empty vanilla pod in a jar then cover it with caster sugar to make your own vanilla sugar.

nectarine and almond tarte tartin

PREP + COOK TIME 50 MINUTES ◆ SERVES 2

5g (¼ ounce) butter

1 tablespoon water

2 tablespoons brown sugar

1 vanilla bean, split lengthways, seeds removed

2 medium nectarines (340g), halved, seeded, cut into thin wedges

1 tablespoon slivered almonds

2 sheets fillo pastry

1 teaspoon skim milk

2 tablespoons fat-free natural yoghurt

1 Preheat oven to 200°C/400°F.

2 Combine butter, the water, sugar and vanilla bean pod and seeds in a small ovenproof frying pan over medium heat; cook, stirring, for 1 minute or until butter has melted and sugar has dissolved.

3 Increase heat to high, add nectarines and nuts; cook, stirring, for 2 minutes or until liquid has thickened slightly. Remove vanilla pod.

4 Meanwhile, brush each pastry sheet on one side with milk, place one pastry sheet on top of the other, brushed-side up; place over nectarines in the pan and carefully tuck pastry in around the edges.

5 Bake for 20 minutes or until pastry is golden and crisp. Carefully turn onto a plate. Cut in half and serve with yoghurt.

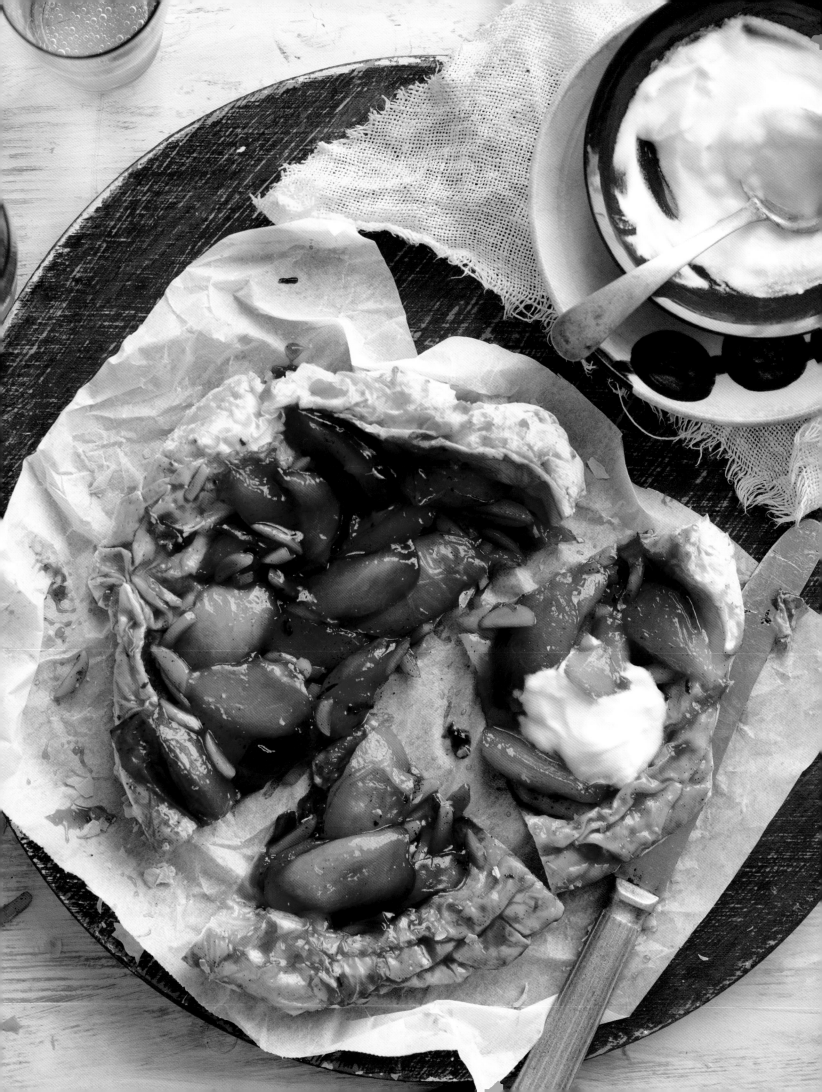

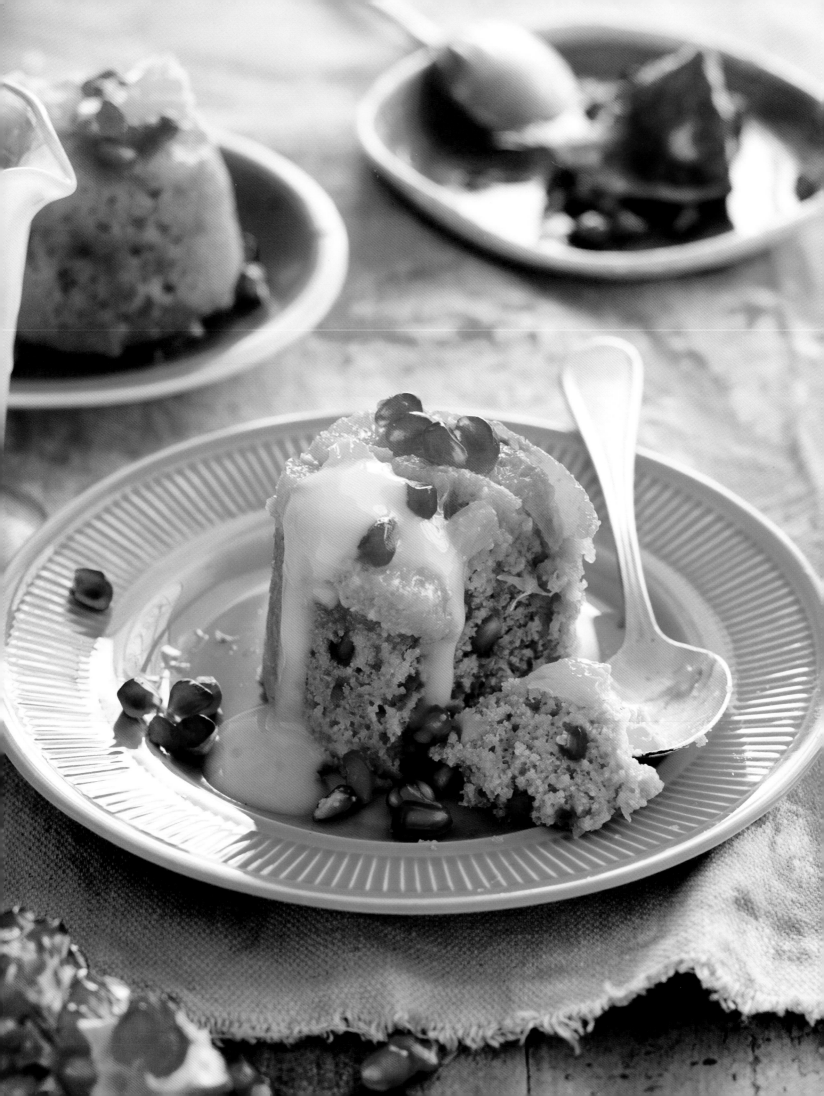

NUTRITIONAL COUNT PER SERVING

● 5.2g total fat   ● 7g protein

● 1g saturated fat   ● 3.5g fibre

● 847kJ (202 cal)   ● 150mg sodium

● 30.7g carbohydrate   ● low GI

orange and pomegranate steamed puddings

PREP + COOK TIME 45 MINUTES ◆ **SERVES** 2

2½ tablespoons brown sugar

½ medium orange (240g), segmented

1 small egg

2½ tablespoons wholemeal self-raising flour

1 tablespoon ground almonds

1 tablespoon orange juice

1 tablespoon fresh pomegranate

1 tablespoon low-fat custard

1 Grease and line base of 2 x ¾-cup (180ml) dariole moulds or ramekins with baking paper.

2 Sprinkle 2 teaspoons of the sugar on the base of the moulds; top with orange segments.

3 Beat remaining sugar and egg in a small bowl with an electric mixer for 2 minutes or until thick and creamy. Fold in remaining ingredients.

4 Divide mixture between moulds, cover with a layer of pleated foil and baking paper; secure with kitchen string.

5 Place puddings in a medium saucepan with enough boiling water to come halfway up the sides of moulds. Cover with a tight fitting lid; simmer for 25 minutes. Stand puddings for 5 minutes. Serve each pudding with 2 teaspoons of custard.

TIP Puddings can be made a day ahead; reheat in a microwave for 15-second bursts until heated through.

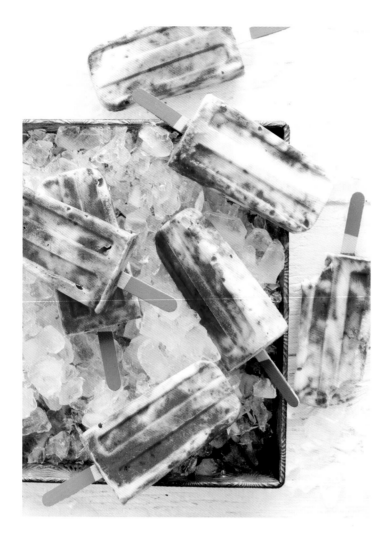

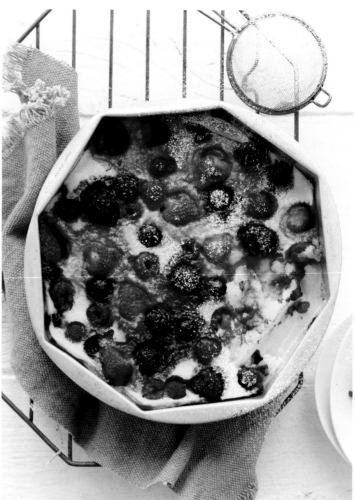

raspberry and vanilla yoghurt ice-blocks

PREP + COOK TIME 25 MINUTES
(+ COOLING & FREEZING) ♦ **MAKES** 14

Combine ¼ cup low-GI cane sugar, 1 split vanilla bean and ¾ cup water in a small saucepan; stir over low heat for 4 minutes or until sugar is dissolved. Bring to the boil without stirring; reduce heat, simmer for 10 minutes or until syrupy. Remove vanilla bean; cool. Blend cooled syrup and 300g (9½ ounces) frozen raspberries until smooth. Very gently swirl in 2⅔ cups low-fat plain yoghurt. Pour into fourteen ⅓-cup (80ml) ice-block moulds. Freeze overnight or until firm.

TIP You could use frozen strawberries, cherries or mango.

mixed berry clafoutis

PREP + COOK TIME 40 MINUTES ♦ **SERVES** 2

Preheat oven to 180°C/350°F. Lightly spray a 2 cup (500ml) shallow baking dish with cooking oil. Whisk 1 egg and ¼ cup plain (all-purpose) flour in a small bowl until combined. Whisk in ¼ cup low-fat milk, 1½ tablespoons caster (superfine) sugar, 1 teaspoon melted butter and 1 teaspoon vanilla extract. Pour into dish. Top with 1 cup frozen mixed berries. Bake for 30 minutes or until mixture is puffed and golden. Dust with ½ teaspoon icing (confectioners') sugar to serve.

TIP You could also serve this with low-GI, low-fat vanilla ice-cream.

NUTRITIONAL COUNT PER SERVING

- **5.6g total fat**
- **2.4g saturated fat**
- **941kJ (245 cal)**
- **32.9g carbohydrate**
- **7.4g protein**
- **3.1g fibre**
- **72mg sodium**
- **medium GI**

NUTRITIONAL COUNT PER SERVING

- **5.6g total fat**
- **2.4g saturated fat**
- **941kJ (245 cal)**
- **32.9g carbohydrate**
- **7.4g protein**
- **3.1g fibre**
- **72mg sodium**
- **medium GI**

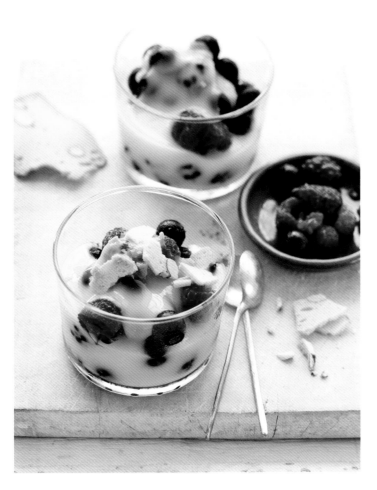

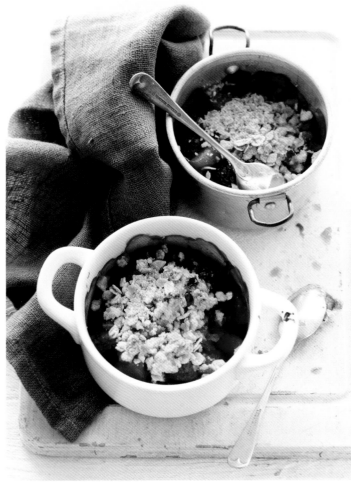

mixed berry fool

PREP TIME 5 MINUTES (+ STANDING) ◆ MAKES 2

Layer 150g (6½ ounces) frozen mixed berries and ⅔-cup low-fat vanilla custard in two ¾-cup (180ml) serving glasses. Sprinkle with 2 finely chopped almond bread. Stand for 20 minutes or until berries have thawed.

TIPS You can thaw the berries in the microwave but assembling this dessert when frozen means you get perfect layers. Assemble it before dinner and it will be ready for dessert. You could make a tropical fool with seeded fresh lychees and fresh passionfruit pulp.

You could also serve this with low-GI, low-fat vanilla ice-cream. This crumble topping would go well with a pear and ginger crumble or apple and raspberry.

apple berry crumble

PREP + COOK TIME 40 MINUTES ◆ MAKES 2

Preheat oven to 200°C/400°F. Peel and coarsely chopped 2 large granny smith apples. Cook apples with 2 tablespoons water in a covered small saucepan over medium heat for 8 minutes or until apples are just tender. Stir through 100g (3 ounces) frozen mixed berries. Divide between two 1-cup (250ml) ovenproof ramekins. Rub 10g (½ ounce) can•ola spread into 1 tablespoon plain (all-purpose) flour in a small bowl until mixture resembles breadcrumbs. Stir in 1 tablespoon rolled oats, 2 teaspoons. low-GI cane sugar and 5 chopped hazelnuts; sprinkle over berry mixture. Bake for 25 minutes or until crumble is golden brown.

NUTRITIONAL COUNT PER SERVING

- 1.9g total fat
- 0.7g saturated fat
- 553kJ (132 cal)
- 22g carbohydrate
- 4.9g protein
- 2.8g fibre
- 50mg sodium
- low GI

NUTRITIONAL COUNT PER SERVING

- 5.7g total fat
- 0.7g saturated fat
- 894kJ (214 cal)
- 35g carbohydrate
- 2.6g protein
- 6.5g fibre
- 24mg sodium
- low GI

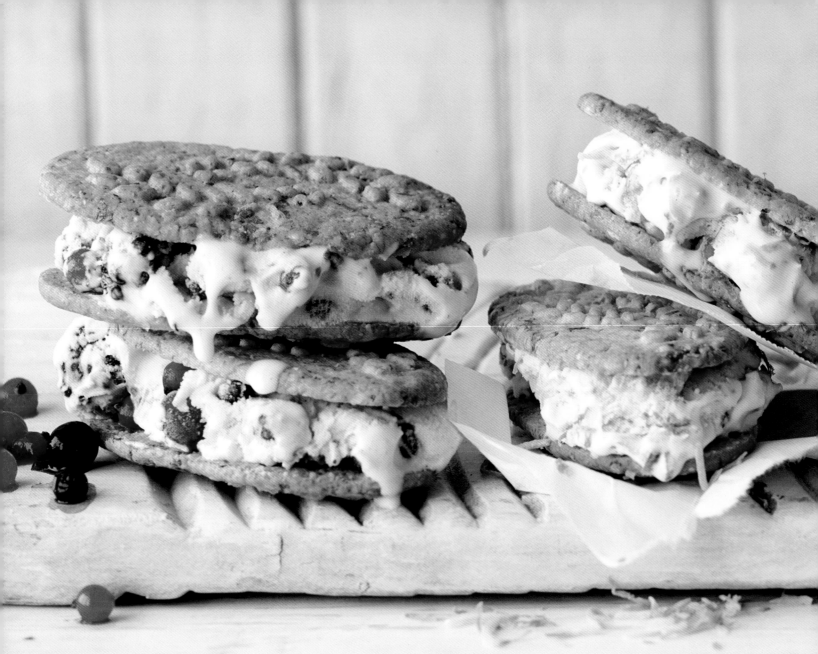

very berry
ice-cream sandwiches

PREP + COOK TIME 15 MINUTES (+ FREEZING) ◆ **SERVES** 2

Combine ¼ cup (35g) mixed frozen berries in a medium bowl. Stand for 10 minutes or until slightly thawed; crush lightly. Stir in ½ cup 97% fat-free no-added sugar vanilla ice-cream. Transfer ice-cream to a freezer-proof container. Freeze for 1 hour or until firm. Sandwich scoops of ice-cream between 4 breakfast biscuits.

TIP We used Belvita Breakfast biscuits. Allow ice-cream to soften slightly before stirring in ingredients.

NUTRITIONAL COUNT PER SERVING

- 4.3g total fat
- 1.3g saturated fat
- 660kJ (158 cal)
- 24.9g carbohydrate
- 3.8g protein
- 1.2g fibre
- 125mg sodium
- low GI

coconut & lime
ice-cream sandwiches

PREP + COOK TIME 10 MINUTES (+ FREEZING) ◆ **SERVES** 2

Combine 2 teaspoons toasted shredded coconut, 1 teaspoon finely grated lime rind and ½ cup 97% fat-free no-added sugar vanilla ice-cream in a medium bowl; stir to combine. Transfer ice-cream to a freezer-proof container. Freeze for 1 hour or until firm. Sandwich scoops of ice-cream between 4 breakfast biscuits.

TIP We used Belvita Breakfast biscuits. Allow ice-cream to soften slightly before stirring in ingredients.

NUTRITIONAL COUNT PER SERVING

- 9.4g total fat
- 1.5g saturated fat
- 1615kJ (386 cal)
- 63g carbohydrate
- 9.3g protein
- 5.3g fibre
- 18mg sodium
- low GI

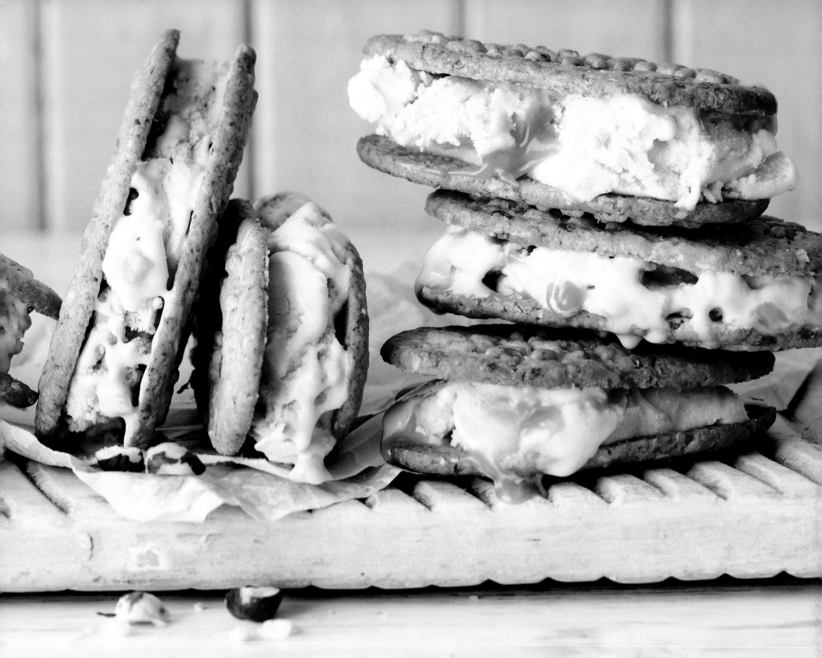

coffee & hazelnut ice-cream sandwiches

PREP + COOK TIME 15 MINUTES (+ FREEZING) ◆ **SERVES** 2

Combine 1 teaspoon cold espresso coffee and 2 teaspoons finely chopped toasted hazelnuts in a medium bowl. Stir in ½ cup 97% fat-free no-added sugar vanilla ice-cream. Transfer ice-cream to a freezer-proof container. Freeze for 1 hour or until firm. Sandwich scoops of ice-cream between 4 breakfast biscuits.

TIP We used Belvita Breakfast biscuits. Allow ice-cream to soften slightly before stirring in ingredients.

NUTRITIONAL COUNT PER SERVING

- 4.9g total fat
- 1.3g saturated fat
- 667kJ (160 cal)
- 24.3g carbohydrate
- 3.6g protein
- 0.9g fibre
- 125mg sodium
- low GI

caramel swirl ice-cream sandwiches

PREP + COOK TIME 10 MINUTES (+ FREEZING) ◆ **SERVES** 2

Combine ½ cup 97% fat-free no-added sugar vanilla ice-cream in a freezer-proof container. Swirl in 2 teaspoons caramel sauce. Freeze for 1 hour or until firm. Sandwich scoops of ice-cream between 4 breakfast biscuits.

TIP We used Belvita Breakfast biscuits. Allow ice-cream to soften slightly before stirring in ingredients.

NUTRITIONAL COUNT PER SERVING

- 4.3g total fat
- 1.3g saturated fat
- 719kJ (172 cal)
- 29g carbohydrate
- 3.6g protein
- 0.8g fibre
- 149mg sodium
- low GI

GLOSSARY

AGAVE SYRUP a sweetener commercially produced from the agave plant in South Africa and Mexico. It is sweeter than sugar, though less viscous, so it dissolves quickly. Agave syrup is sold in light, amber, dark, and raw varieties.

ALL-BRAN CEREAL a low-fat, high-fibre breakfast cereal based on wheat bran.

BAKING POWDER a raising agent consisting mainly of two parts cream of tartar to one part bicarbonate of soda (baking soda).

BASIL, THAI (also horapa); different from sweet basil in both look and taste, having smaller leaves and purplish stems and a slight aniseed taste.

BEANS
black also known as turtle beans or black kidney beans; an earthy-flavoured bean completely different from the better-known chinese black beans (which are fermented soya beans).
broad also known as fava, windsor and horse beans. Fresh and frozen forms should be peeled twice (discarding both the outer long green pod and the beige-green tough inner shell).
cannellini small white bean similar in appearance and flavour to great northern, navy and haricot beans — all of which can be substituted for the other. Available dried or canned.
kidney medium-sized red bean, slightly floury in texture yet sweet in flavour.
sprouts also known as bean shoots; tender new growths of assorted beans and seeds grown for consumption as sprouts. The most readily available are mung bean, soya bean, alfalfa and snow pea sprouts.
white in this book, 'white beans', is a generic term we use for cannellini, great northern, haricot or navy beans, all of which can be substituted for the other.

BICARBONATE OF SODA also known as baking or carb soda; is used as a leavening agent in baking.

BUK CHOY also known as bok choy, pak choi, chinese white cabbage or chinese chard; has a fresh, mild mustard taste. Baby buk choy, also known as pak kat farang or shanghai bok choy, is much smaller and more tender than buk choy.

BUTTERMILK originally the term given to the slightly sour liquid left after butter was churned from cream, today it is made similarly to yogurt. Sold alongside all fresh milk products in supermarkets; despite he implication of its name, it is low in fat.

CAVOLO NERO also known as tuscan cabbage or tuscan black cabbage. It has long, narrow, wrinkled leaves and a rich and astringent, mild cabbage flavour. It doesn't lose its volume like silver beet or spinach when cooked, but it does need longer cooking. It is a member of the kale family; if you can't find it use silver beet (swiss chard) or cabbage instead.

CHEESE
cottage fresh, white, unripened curd cheese with a grainy consistency and a fat content between 5% and 15%.
cream commonly known as Philadelphia or Philly; a soft cows'-milk cheese with a fat content of at least 33%. Also available as spreadable light cream cheese, a blend of cottage and cream cheeses with a fat content of 21%.
goat made from goats' milk, has an earthy, strong taste; available in soft and firm textures, in various shapes and sizes, and sometimes rolled in ash or herbs.
mozzarella a soft, spun-curd cheese. It has a low melting point and an elastic texture when heated; used to add texture rather than flavour. A favourite cheese for pizza.
parmesan also known as parmigiano, parmesan is a hard, grainy cows'-milk cheese. The curd is salted in brine for a month before being aged for up to two years in humid conditions.
ricotta the name for this soft, white, cows'-milk cheese roughly translates as 'cooked again'. It's made from whey, a by-product of other cheese-making, to which fresh milk and acid are added.
tasty a matured cheddar; use an aged, strongly-flavoured, hard variety.

CHICKPEAS also called garbanzos, hummus or channa; an irregularly round, sandy-coloured legume.

CHILLI available in many different types and sizes. Use rubber gloves when seeding and chopping fresh chillies as they can burn your skin. Removing seeds and membranes lessens the heat level.
flakes, dried deep-red, dehydrated chilli slices and whole seeds.
long green or red available both fresh and dried; a generic term used for moderately hot, long (about 6cm to 8cm), thin chillies.
red thai also known as 'scuds'; small, very hot and bright red in colour.

CHINESE FIVE-SPICE POWDER a fragrant mixture of ground cinnamon, cloves, star anise, sichuan pepper and fennel seeds.

CHOY SUM also known as pakaukeo or flowering cabbage, a member of the buk choy family; easy to identify with its long stems, light green leaves and yellow flowers. Is eaten, stems and all, steamed or stir-fried.

CORIANDER also known as pak chee, cilantro or chinese parsley; bright-green leafy herb with a pungent flavour. Both the stems and roots of coriander are used; wash well before using. Is also available ground or as seeds; these should not be substituted for fresh as the tastes are completely different.

CORNFLOUR also known as cornstarch; used as a thickening agent in cooking. Buy 100% corn (maize) cornflour, as wheaten cornflour is made from wheat rather than corn and contains some gluten.

CREAM we used fresh cream, also known as pouring or pure cream, unless otherwise stated. It has no additives unlike thickened cream. Minimum fat content 35%.
sour a thick, cultured soured cream. Minimum fat content 35%.
thickened a whipping cream containing a thickener. Minimum fat content 35%.

DAIKON also known as giant white radish. Used extensively in Japanese cooking; has a sweet, fresh flavour without the bite of the common red radish.

FENNEL also known as finocchio or anise; a white to very pale green-white, firm, crisp, roundish vegetable about 8cm-12cm in diameter. The bulb has a slightly sweet, anise flavour but the leaves have a much stronger taste. Also the name given to dried seeds having a licorice flavour.

FLAT-LEAF PARSLEY also known as continental parsley or italian parsley.

FLOUR
buckwheat a herb in the same plant family as rhubarb; not a cereal so it is gluten-free.
plain an all-purpose flour made from wheat.
rice a very fine flour, made from ground white rice.
self-raising plain flour sifted with baking powder in the proportion of 1 cup flour to 2 teaspoons baking powder. Also called self-rising flour.
spelt very similar to wheat, but has a slightly nuttier, sweeter flavour. Spelt flour contains gluten.
wholemeal milled from whole wheat grain (bran, germ and endosperm).

GAI LAN also known as chinese broccoli, gai larn, kanah, gai lum and chinese kale; appreciated more for its stems than its coarse leaves.

HARISSA a hot Moroccan sauce or paste made from dried chillies, cumin, garlic, oil and caraway seeds. The paste, available in a tube, is very hot and should not be used in large amounts; bottled harissa sauce is milder, but is still hot. If you have a low heat-level tolerance, you may find any recipe containing harissa too hot to tolerate. Available from supermarkets and Middle-Eastern grocery stores.

KAFFIR LIME LEAVES also known as bai magrood, look like two glossy dark green leaves joined end to end, forming a rounded hourglass shape. Dried leaves are less potent so double the number if using them as a substitute for fresh. A strip of fresh lime peel may be substituted for each kaffir lime leaf.

MAPLE SYRUP a thin syrup distilled from the sap of the maple tree. Maple-flavoured or pancake syrup is not an adequate substitute for the real thing.

MISO Japan's famous bean paste made from fermented soya beans and rice, rye or barley. White miso tends to have a sweeter and somewhat less salty flavour than the darker red miso. Dissolve miso in a little water before adding. Keeps well refrigerated.

MOUNTAIN BREAD a thin, soft-textured bread, that can be rolled up and filled.

MUSHROOM
cup a common white mushroom picked just as the veil, or underside, begins to open around the stem. Has a full-bodied flavour and firm texture.
enoki clumps of long, spaghetti-like stems with tiny, snowy white caps.
flat large, flat mushrooms with a rich earthy flavour. They are sometimes misnamed field mushrooms, which are wild mushrooms.
porcini, dried the richest flavoured mushrooms; also known as cèpes. Have a strong nutty flavour, so only small amounts are required. Rehydrate before use.
shiitake when fresh are also known as chinese black, forest or golden oak mushrooms; although cultivated, they have the earthiness and taste of wild mushrooms. Are large and meaty.
swiss brown also called roman or cremini; are light-to-dark brown in colour with a full-bodied flavour.

OIL, GRAPE SEED is a good-quality, neutral vegetable oil pressed from grape seeds.

PAPRIKA ground dried sweet red capsicum (bell pepper); there are many grades and types available.

POMEGRANATE MOLASSES thick, tangy syrup made by boiling pomegranate juice into a sticky, syrupy consistency. Available from Middle Eastern food stores, specialty food shops and delis.

POTATO, BABY NEW also known as chats; not a separate variety but an early harvest with very thin skin.

PROSCIUTTO a dry-cured Italian ham. Available as crudo (raw) and cotto (cooked).

QUINOA (keen-wa) the seed of a leafy plant similar to spinach. It has a delicate, slightly nutty taste and chewy texture. Its cooking qualities are similar to that of rice. You can buy it in most health-food stores; it spoils easily, so keep it sealed in a glass jar in the fridge. Quinoa flakes are rolled and flattened grains.

RHUBARB has thick, celery-like stalks that can reach up to 60cm long; the stalks are the only edible portion of the plant as the leaves contain a toxic substance.

RICE
basmati a white, fragrant long-grained rice. Wash well before cooking.
brown basmati has more fibre and a stronger flavour than white basmati, but it takes twice as long to cook.
microwave milled, cooked then dried rice. Pre-cooked rice is more porous, so that steam can penetrate the grain and rehydrate it in a short time.

RICE NOODLES, DRIED made from rice flour and water, available flat and wide or very thin (vermicelli). Should be soaked in boiling water to soften. Also known as rice stick noodles.

RISONI a small, rice-shaped pasta.

ROLLED OATS oat groats (oats that have been husked) steam-softened, flattened with rollers, then dried and packaged.

SASHIMI GRADE SALMON use the freshest, sashimi-quality fish you can find. Raw fish sold as sashimi has to meet stringent guidelines regarding its handling and treatment after leaving the water. Seek local advice from authorities before eating any raw seafood.

SAUCE
fish made from pulverised fermented fish, most often anchovies. Has a pungent smell and strong taste; use sparingly.

hoisin a thick, sweet and spicy chinese paste made from salted fermented soya beans, onions and garlic.

oyster Asian in origin; a rich, brown sauce made from oysters and their brine, cooked with soy sauce, and thickened with starch.
soy also known as sieu, is made from fermented soya beans. Several variations are available in most supermarkets and Asian food stores.
sweet chilli a comparatively mild, thai-type sauce made from red chillies, sugar, garlic and vinegar.

SEMOLINA made from durum (hard) wheat milled into textured granules.

SHALLOT also french or golden shallots or eschalots; small, elongated, brown-skinned members of the onion family. Grows in tight clusters similar to garlic.

SNOW PEAS also called mange tout (eat all). Snow pea tendrils, the growing shoots of the plant, are sold by greengrocers. Snow pea sprouts tender new growths of snow peas; also known as mange tout.

SUGAR
brown a soft, finely granulated sugar retaining molasses for its characteristic colour and flavour.
caster also known as superfine or finely granulated table sugar.
icing also known as confectioners' sugar or powdered sugar; granulated sugar crushed with a small amount of cornflour.
low-GI cane a molasses extract is sprayed onto raw sugar, increasing the time it takes to digest the sugar, resulting in a slower release of energy.

SULTANAS also known as golden raisins.

SUMAC a purple-red, astringent spice ground from berries grown on shrubs that flourish around the Mediterranean; adds a tart, lemony flavour to foods.

TURMERIC a member of the ginger family, its root is dried and ground, resulting in the rich yellow powder that gives many Indian dishes their characteristic colour. It is intensely pungent in taste, but not hot.

VINEGAR
balsamic made from Trebbiano grapes; has a deep rich brown colour with a sweet and sour flavour.
red wine based on fermented red wine.

WASABI an Asian horseradish used to make the pungent, green-coloured sauce traditionally served with Japanese raw fish dishes; sold in powdered or paste form.

CONVERSION CHART

measures

One Australian metric measuring cup holds approximately 250ml; one Australian metric tablespoon holds 20ml; one Australian metric teaspoon holds 5ml.
The difference between one country's measuring cups and anothers is within a two- or three-teaspoon variance, and will not affect your cooking results.
North America, New Zealand and the United Kingdom use a 15ml tablespoon.
All cup and spoon measurements are level. The most accurate way of measuring dry ingredients is to weigh them. When measuring liquids, use a clear glass or plastic jug with the metric markings.
The imperial measurements used in these recipes are approximate only. Do not mix measurements; use either all metric or all imperial. Measurements for cake pans are approximate only. Using same-shaped cake pans of a similar size should not affect the outcome of your baking. We measure the inside top of the cake pan to determine sizes.
We use large eggs with an average weight of 60g.

dry measures

metric	imperial
15g	½oz
30g	1oz
60g	2oz
90g	3oz
125g	4oz (¼lb)
155g	5oz
185g	6oz
220g	7oz
250g	8oz (½lb)
280g	9oz
315g	10oz
345g	11oz
375g	12oz (¾lb)
410g	13oz
440g	14oz
470g	15oz
500g	16oz (1lb)
750g	24oz (1½lb)
1kg	32oz (2lb)

liquid measures

metric	imperial
30ml	1 fluid oz
60ml	2 fluid oz
100ml	3 fluid oz
125ml	4 fluid oz
150ml	5 fluid oz
190ml	6 fluid oz
250ml	8 fluid oz
300ml	10 fluid oz
500ml	16 fluid oz
600ml	20 fluid oz
1000ml (1 litre)	1¾ pints

length measures

metric	imperial
3mm	⅛in
6mm	¼in
1cm	½in
2cm	¾in
2.5cm	1in
5cm	2in
6cm	2½in
8cm	3in
10cm	4in
13cm	5in
15cm	6in
18cm	7in
20cm	8in
22cm	9in
25cm	10in
28cm	11in
30cm	12in (1ft)

oven temperatures

The oven temperatures in this book are for conventional ovens;
if you have a fan-forced oven, decrease the temperature by 10-20 degrees.

	°C (CELSIUS)	°F (FAHRENHEIT)
Very slow	120	250
Slow	150	300
Moderately slow	160	325
Moderate	180	350
Moderately hot	200	400
Hot	220	425
Very hot	240	475

INDEX